THIS Intermittent Fasting JOURNAL AND TI
HELP You CRUSH ALL YOUR health and we......
TO FASTING, WHETHER IT BE FOR weight loss, autophagy, aging,
OR ALL THE many other benefits THAT COME WITH
INTERMITTENT FASTING.

In this journal you can....

TRACK DAILY FASTS FOR AN ENTIRE YEAR

LOG YOUR MOODS

KEEP TRACK OF YOUR WATER INTAKE

WEEKLY BODY MEASUREMENTS

LOG WEIGHT LOSS, GAIN, OR MAINTENANCE

RECORD STRUGGLES & VICTORIES WITH EXTRA SPACE FOR

PERSONAL NOTES

AND FIND INSPIRATIONAL QUOTES TO REFLECT ON WEEKLY

---

copyright © 2020 by Fasting to Fab Journals

Daily Fasting Tracker

	1AM	2AM	3AM	4AM	5AM	6AM	7AM	8AM	9AM	10AM	11AM	12PM	1PM	2PM	3PM	4PM	5PM	6PM	7PM	8PM	9PM	10PM	11PM	12AM
Monday	○	○	○	○	○	○	○	○	○	○	○	○	○	○	○	○	○	○	○	○	○	○	○	○
Tuesday	○	○	○	○	○	○	○	○	○	○	○	○	○	○	○	○	○	○	○	○	○	○	○	○
Wednesday	○	○	○	○	○	○	○	○	○	○	○	○	○	○	○	○	○	○	○	○	○	○	○	○
Thursday	○	○	○	○	○	○	○	○	○	○	○	○	○	○	○	○	○	○	○	○	○	○	○	○
Friday	○	○	○	○	○	○	○	○	○	○	○	○	○	○	○	○	○	○	○	○	○	○	○	○
Saturday	○	○	○	○	○	○	○	○	○	○	○	○	○	○	○	○	○	○	○	○	○	○	○	○
Sunday	○	○	○	○	○	○	○	○	○	○	○	○	○	○	○	○	○	○	○	○	○	○	○	○

Mood

MON
TUE
WED
THU
FRI
SAT
SUN

Daily Water Log

MON
TUES
WED
THU
FRI
SAT
SUN

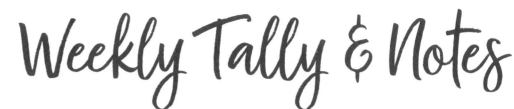

Weekly Tally & Notes

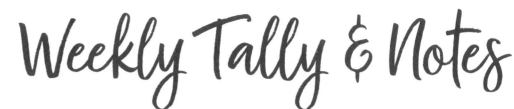

bust —————
upper arm ———
waist —————
————— hips
upper leg ————

Body Measurements:

BUST _____
UPPER ARM _____
WAIST _____
HIPS _____
UPPER LEG _____

Weekly Weight Tracker

CURRENT WEIGHT _____
GOAL WEIGHT _____

STRUGGLES

VICTORIES

Notes:

Set goals and crush them.

Daily Fasting Tracker

	1AM	2AM	3AM	4AM	5AM	6AM	7AM	8AM	9AM	10AM	11AM	12PM	1PM	2PM	3PM	4PM	5PM	6PM	7PM	8PM	9PM	10PM	11PM	12AM
Monday	○	○	○	○	○	○	○	○	○	○	○	○	○	○	○	○	○	○	○	○	○	○	○	○
Tuesday	○	○	○	○	○	○	○	○	○	○	○	○	○	○	○	○	○	○	○	○	○	○	○	○
Wednesday	○	○	○	○	○	○	○	○	○	○	○	○	○	○	○	○	○	○	○	○	○	○	○	○
Thursday	○	○	○	○	○	○	○	○	○	○	○	○	○	○	○	○	○	○	○	○	○	○	○	○
Friday	○	○	○	○	○	○	○	○	○	○	○	○	○	○	○	○	○	○	○	○	○	○	○	○
Saturday	○	○	○	○	○	○	○	○	○	○	○	○	○	○	○	○	○	○	○	○	○	○	○	○
Sunday	○	○	○	○	○	○	○	○	○	○	○	○	○	○	○	○	○	○	○	○	○	○	○	○

Mood

MON
TUE
WED
THU
FRI
SAT
SUN

Daily Water Log

MON	🌢 🌢 🌢 🌢 🌢 🌢 🌢 🌢
TUES	🌢 🌢 🌢 🌢 🌢 🌢 🌢 🌢
WED	🌢 🌢 🌢 🌢 🌢 🌢 🌢 🌢
THU	🌢 🌢 🌢 🌢 🌢 🌢 🌢 🌢
FRI	🌢 🌢 🌢 🌢 🌢 🌢 🌢 🌢
SAT	🌢 🌢 🌢 🌢 🌢 🌢 🌢 🌢
SUN	🌢 🌢 🌢 🌢 🌢 🌢 🌢 🌢

Weekly Tally & Notes

bust

upper arm

waist

hips

upper leg

Body Measurements:

BUST _____
UPPER ARM _____
WAIST _____
HIPS _____
UPPER LEG _____

Weekly Weight Tracker

CURRENT WEIGHT _____
GOAL WEIGHT _____

STRUGGLES

VICTORIES

Notes:

Take a step towards the person you want to be.

Daily Fasting Tracker

	1AM	2AM	3AM	4AM	5AM	6AM	7AM	8AM	9AM	10AM	11AM	12PM	1PM	2PM	3PM	4PM	5PM	6PM	7PM	8PM	9PM	10PM	11PM	12AM
Monday	○	○	○	○	○	○	○	○	○	○	○	○	○	○	○	○	○	○	○	○	○	○	○	○
Tuesday	○	○	○	○	○	○	○	○	○	○	○	○	○	○	○	○	○	○	○	○	○	○	○	○
Wednesday	○	○	○	○	○	○	○	○	○	○	○	○	○	○	○	○	○	○	○	○	○	○	○	○
Thursday	○	○	○	○	○	○	○	○	○	○	○	○	○	○	○	○	○	○	○	○	○	○	○	○
Friday	○	○	○	○	○	○	○	○	○	○	○	○	○	○	○	○	○	○	○	○	○	○	○	○
Saturday	○	○	○	○	○	○	○	○	○	○	○	○	○	○	○	○	○	○	○	○	○	○	○	○
Sunday	○	○	○	○	○	○	○	○	○	○	○	○	○	○	○	○	○	○	○	○	○	○	○	○

Mood

MON
TUE
WED
THU
FRI
SAT
SUN

Daily Water Log

MON
TUES
WED
THU
FRI
SAT
SUN

Weekly Tally & Notes

bust
upper arm
waist
hips
upper leg

Body Measurements:

BUST _____
UPPER ARM _____
WAIST _____
HIPS _____
UPPER LEG _____

Weekly Weight Tracker

CURRENT WEIGHT _____
GOAL WEIGHT _____

STRUGGLES

VICTORIES

Notes:

If you can't stop thinking about it, don't stop working for it.

Daily Fasting Tracker

	1AM	2AM	3AM	4AM	5AM	6AM	7AM	8AM	9AM	10AM	11AM	12PM	1PM	2PM	3PM	4PM	5PM	6PM	7PM	8PM	9PM	10PM	11PM	12AM
Monday	○	○	○	○	○	○	○	○	○	○	○	○	○	○	○	○	○	○	○	○	○	○	○	○
Tuesday	○	○	○	○	○	○	○	○	○	○	○	○	○	○	○	○	○	○	○	○	○	○	○	○
Wednesday	○	○	○	○	○	○	○	○	○	○	○	○	○	○	○	○	○	○	○	○	○	○	○	○
Thursday	○	○	○	○	○	○	○	○	○	○	○	○	○	○	○	○	○	○	○	○	○	○	○	○
Friday	○	○	○	○	○	○	○	○	○	○	○	○	○	○	○	○	○	○	○	○	○	○	○	○
Saturday	○	○	○	○	○	○	○	○	○	○	○	○	○	○	○	○	○	○	○	○	○	○	○	○
Sunday	○	○	○	○	○	○	○	○	○	○	○	○	○	○	○	○	○	○	○	○	○	○	○	○

Mood

MON
TUE
WED
THU
FRI
SAT
SUN

Daily Water Log

MON
TUES
WED
THU
FRI
SAT
SUN

Weekly Tally & Notes

bust

upper arm

waist

hips

upper leg

Body Measurements:

BUST _____
UPPER ARM _____
WAIST _____
HIPS _____
UPPER LEG _____

Weekly Weight Tracker

CURRENT WEIGHT _____
GOAL WEIGHT _____

STRUGGLES

VICTORIES

Notes:

Be Focused. Be Persistent. Never Quit

Daily Fasting Tracker

	1AM	2AM	3AM	4AM	5AM	6AM	7AM	8AM	9AM	10AM	11AM	12PM	1PM	2PM	3PM	4PM	5PM	6PM	7PM	8PM	9PM	10PM	11PM	12AM
Monday	○	○	○	○	○	○	○	○	○	○	○	○	○	○	○	○	○	○	○	○	○	○	○	○
Tuesday	○	○	○	○	○	○	○	○	○	○	○	○	○	○	○	○	○	○	○	○	○	○	○	○
Wednesday	○	○	○	○	○	○	○	○	○	○	○	○	○	○	○	○	○	○	○	○	○	○	○	○
Thursday	○	○	○	○	○	○	○	○	○	○	○	○	○	○	○	○	○	○	○	○	○	○	○	○
Friday	○	○	○	○	○	○	○	○	○	○	○	○	○	○	○	○	○	○	○	○	○	○	○	○
Saturday	○	○	○	○	○	○	○	○	○	○	○	○	○	○	○	○	○	○	○	○	○	○	○	○
Sunday	○	○	○	○	○	○	○	○	○	○	○	○	○	○	○	○	○	○	○	○	○	○	○	○

Mood

MON
TUE
WED
THU
FRI
SAT
SUN

Daily Water Log

MON	◌ ◌ ◌ ◌ ◌ ◌ ◌ ◌
TUES	◌ ◌ ◌ ◌ ◌ ◌ ◌ ◌
WED	◌ ◌ ◌ ◌ ◌ ◌ ◌ ◌
THU	◌ ◌ ◌ ◌ ◌ ◌ ◌ ◌
FRI	◌ ◌ ◌ ◌ ◌ ◌ ◌ ◌
SAT	◌ ◌ ◌ ◌ ◌ ◌ ◌ ◌
SUN	◌ ◌ ◌ ◌ ◌ ◌ ◌ ◌

Weekly Tally & Notes

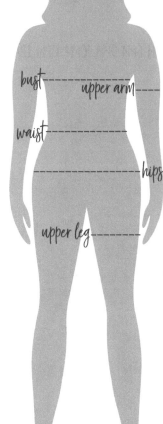

bust
upper arm
waist
hips
upper leg

Body Measurements:

BUST _____
UPPER ARM _____
WAIST _____
HIPS _____
UPPER LEG _____

Weekly Weight Tracker

CURRENT WEIGHT _____
GOAL WEIGHT _____

STRUGGLES

VICTORIES

Notes:

There are seven days in a week and someday isn't one of them.

WEEK SIX
FASTING SCHEDULE : __/__

Daily Fasting Tracker

	1AM	2AM	3AM	4AM	5AM	6AM	7AM	8AM	9AM	10AM	11AM	12PM	1PM	2PM	3PM	4PM	5PM	6PM	7PM	8PM	9PM	10PM	11PM	12AM
Monday	○	○	○	○	○	○	○	○	○	○	○	○	○	○	○	○	○	○	○	○	○	○	○	○
Tuesday	○	○	○	○	○	○	○	○	○	○	○	○	○	○	○	○	○	○	○	○	○	○	○	○
Wednesday	○	○	○	○	○	○	○	○	○	○	○	○	○	○	○	○	○	○	○	○	○	○	○	○
Thursday	○	○	○	○	○	○	○	○	○	○	○	○	○	○	○	○	○	○	○	○	○	○	○	○
Friday	○	○	○	○	○	○	○	○	○	○	○	○	○	○	○	○	○	○	○	○	○	○	○	○
Saturday	○	○	○	○	○	○	○	○	○	○	○	○	○	○	○	○	○	○	○	○	○	○	○	○
Sunday	○	○	○	○	○	○	○	○	○	○	○	○	○	○	○	○	○	○	○	○	○	○	○	○

Mood

Daily Water Log

Weekly Tally & Notes

Body Measurements:

BUST _____

UPPER ARM _____

WAIST _____

HIPS _____

UPPER LEG _____

Weekly Weight Tracker

CURRENT WEIGHT _____

GOAL WEIGHT _____

STRUGGLES

VICTORIES

Notes:

bust

upper arm

waist

hips

upper leg

Dream big. Work hard.
Make it happen.

Daily Fasting Tracker

	1AM	2AM	3AM	4AM	5AM	6AM	7AM	8AM	9AM	10AM	11AM	12PM	1PM	2PM	3PM	4PM	5PM	6PM	7PM	8PM	9PM	10PM	11PM	12AM
Monday	○	○	○	○	○	○	○	○	○	○	○	○	○	○	○	○	○	○	○	○	○	○	○	○
Tuesday	○	○	○	○	○	○	○	○	○	○	○	○	○	○	○	○	○	○	○	○	○	○	○	○
Wednesday	○	○	○	○	○	○	○	○	○	○	○	○	○	○	○	○	○	○	○	○	○	○	○	○
Thursday	○	○	○	○	○	○	○	○	○	○	○	○	○	○	○	○	○	○	○	○	○	○	○	○
Friday	○	○	○	○	○	○	○	○	○	○	○	○	○	○	○	○	○	○	○	○	○	○	○	○
Saturday	○	○	○	○	○	○	○	○	○	○	○	○	○	○	○	○	○	○	○	○	○	○	○	○
Sunday	○	○	○	○	○	○	○	○	○	○	○	○	○	○	○	○	○	○	○	○	○	○	○	○

Mood

MON
TUE
WED
THU
FRI
SAT
SUN

Daily Water Log

MON	◇ ◇ ◇ ◇ ◇ ◇ ◇ ◇
TUES	◇ ◇ ◇ ◇ ◇ ◇ ◇ ◇
WED	◇ ◇ ◇ ◇ ◇ ◇ ◇ ◇
THU	◇ ◇ ◇ ◇ ◇ ◇ ◇ ◇
FRI	◇ ◇ ◇ ◇ ◇ ◇ ◇ ◇
SAT	◇ ◇ ◇ ◇ ◇ ◇ ◇ ◇
SUN	◇ ◇ ◇ ◇ ◇ ◇ ◇ ◇

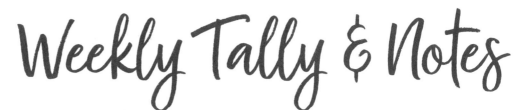

Weekly Tally & Notes

bust
upper arm
waist
hips
upper leg

Body Measurements:

BUST _____
UPPER ARM _____
WAIST _____
HIPS _____
UPPER LEG _____

Weekly Weight Tracker

CURRENT WEIGHT _____
GOAL WEIGHT _____

STRUGGLES

VICTORIES

Notes:

You only fail if you give up.

Daily Fasting Tracker

	1AM	2AM	3AM	4AM	5AM	6AM	7AM	8AM	9AM	10AM	11AM	12PM	1PM	2PM	3PM	4PM	5PM	6PM	7PM	8PM	9PM	10PM	11PM	12AM
Monday	○	○	○	○	○	○	○	○	○	○	○	○	○	○	○	○	○	○	○	○	○	○	○	○
Tuesday	○	○	○	○	○	○	○	○	○	○	○	○	○	○	○	○	○	○	○	○	○	○	○	○
Wednesday	○	○	○	○	○	○	○	○	○	○	○	○	○	○	○	○	○	○	○	○	○	○	○	○
Thursday	○	○	○	○	○	○	○	○	○	○	○	○	○	○	○	○	○	○	○	○	○	○	○	○
Friday	○	○	○	○	○	○	○	○	○	○	○	○	○	○	○	○	○	○	○	○	○	○	○	○
Saturday	○	○	○	○	○	○	○	○	○	○	○	○	○	○	○	○	○	○	○	○	○	○	○	○
Sunday	○	○	○	○	○	○	○	○	○	○	○	○	○	○	○	○	○	○	○	○	○	○	○	○

Mood

MON
TUE
WED
THU
FRI
SAT
SUN

Daily Water Log

MON
TUES
WED
THU
FRI
SAT
SUN

Weekly Tally & Notes

bust
upper arm
waist
hips
upper leg

Body Measurements:

BUST _____
UPPER ARM _____
WAIST _____
HIPS _____
UPPER LEG _____

Weekly Weight Tracker

CURRENT WEIGHT _____
GOAL WEIGHT _____

STRUGGLES

VICTORIES

Notes:

You are entirely up to you.

Daily Fasting Tracker

	1AM	2AM	3AM	4AM	5AM	6AM	7AM	8AM	9AM	10AM	11AM	12PM	1PM	2PM	3PM	4PM	5PM	6PM	7PM	8PM	9PM	10PM	11PM	12AM
Monday	○	○	○	○	○	○	○	○	○	○	○	○	○	○	○	○	○	○	○	○	○	○	○	○
Tuesday	○	○	○	○	○	○	○	○	○	○	○	○	○	○	○	○	○	○	○	○	○	○	○	○
Wednesday	○	○	○	○	○	○	○	○	○	○	○	○	○	○	○	○	○	○	○	○	○	○	○	○
Thursday	○	○	○	○	○	○	○	○	○	○	○	○	○	○	○	○	○	○	○	○	○	○	○	○
Friday	○	○	○	○	○	○	○	○	○	○	○	○	○	○	○	○	○	○	○	○	○	○	○	○
Saturday	○	○	○	○	○	○	○	○	○	○	○	○	○	○	○	○	○	○	○	○	○	○	○	○
Sunday	○	○	○	○	○	○	○	○	○	○	○	○	○	○	○	○	○	○	○	○	○	○	○	○

Mood

MON
TUE
WED
THU
FRI
SAT
SUN

Daily Water Log

MON	○ ○ ○ ○ ○ ○ ○ ○
TUES	○ ○ ○ ○ ○ ○ ○ ○
WED	○ ○ ○ ○ ○ ○ ○ ○
THU	○ ○ ○ ○ ○ ○ ○ ○
FRI	○ ○ ○ ○ ○ ○ ○ ○
SAT	○ ○ ○ ○ ○ ○ ○ ○
SUN	○ ○ ○ ○ ○ ○ ○ ○

Weekly Tally & Notes

bust----------
upper arm----------
waist----------
hips
upper leg----------

Body Measurements:

BUST _____
UPPER ARM _____
WAIST _____
HIPS _____
UPPER LEG _____

Weekly Weight Tracker

CURRENT WEIGHT _____
GOAL WEIGHT _____

STRUGGLES

VICTORIES

Notes:

Doubt kills more dreams than failure ever will.

Daily Fasting Tracker

	1AM	2AM	3AM	4AM	5AM	6AM	7AM	8AM	9AM	10AM	11AM	12PM	1PM	2PM	3PM	4PM	5PM	6PM	7PM	8PM	9PM	10PM	11PM	12AM
Monday	○	○	○	○	○	○	○	○	○	○	○	○	○	○	○	○	○	○	○	○	○	○	○	○
Tuesday	○	○	○	○	○	○	○	○	○	○	○	○	○	○	○	○	○	○	○	○	○	○	○	○
Wednesday	○	○	○	○	○	○	○	○	○	○	○	○	○	○	○	○	○	○	○	○	○	○	○	○
Thursday	○	○	○	○	○	○	○	○	○	○	○	○	○	○	○	○	○	○	○	○	○	○	○	○
Friday	○	○	○	○	○	○	○	○	○	○	○	○	○	○	○	○	○	○	○	○	○	○	○	○
Saturday	○	○	○	○	○	○	○	○	○	○	○	○	○	○	○	○	○	○	○	○	○	○	○	○
Sunday	○	○	○	○	○	○	○	○	○	○	○	○	○	○	○	○	○	○	○	○	○	○	○	○

Mood

MON
TUE
WED
THU
FRI
SAT
SUN

Daily Water Log

MON
TUES
WED
THU
FRI
SAT
SUN

Weekly Tally & Notes

bust
upper arm
waist
hips
upper leg

Body Measurements:

BUST _____
UPPER ARM _____
WAIST _____
HIPS _____
UPPER LEG _____

Weekly Weight Tracker

CURRENT WEIGHT _____
GOAL WEIGHT _____

STRUGGLES

VICTORIES

Notes:

Be you. Do you. For you.

Daily Fasting Tracker

	1AM	2AM	3AM	4AM	5AM	6AM	7AM	8AM	9AM	10AM	11AM	12PM	1PM	2PM	3PM	4PM	5PM	6PM	7PM	8PM	9PM	10PM	11PM	12AM
Monday	○	○	○	○	○	○	○	○	○	○	○	○	○	○	○	○	○	○	○	○	○	○	○	○
Tuesday	○	○	○	○	○	○	○	○	○	○	○	○	○	○	○	○	○	○	○	○	○	○	○	○
Wednesday	○	○	○	○	○	○	○	○	○	○	○	○	○	○	○	○	○	○	○	○	○	○	○	○
Thursday	○	○	○	○	○	○	○	○	○	○	○	○	○	○	○	○	○	○	○	○	○	○	○	○
Friday	○	○	○	○	○	○	○	○	○	○	○	○	○	○	○	○	○	○	○	○	○	○	○	○
Saturday	○	○	○	○	○	○	○	○	○	○	○	○	○	○	○	○	○	○	○	○	○	○	○	○
Sunday	○	○	○	○	○	○	○	○	○	○	○	○	○	○	○	○	○	○	○	○	○	○	○	○

Mood

MON
TUE
WED
THU
FRI
SAT
SUN

Daily Water Log

MON	🜄 🜄 🜄 🜄 🜄 🜄 🜄 🜄
TUES	🜄 🜄 🜄 🜄 🜄 🜄 🜄 🜄
WED	🜄 🜄 🜄 🜄 🜄 🜄 🜄 🜄
THU	🜄 🜄 🜄 🜄 🜄 🜄 🜄 🜄
FRI	🜄 🜄 🜄 🜄 🜄 🜄 🜄 🜄
SAT	🜄 🜄 🜄 🜄 🜄 🜄 🜄 🜄
SUN	🜄 🜄 🜄 🜄 🜄 🜄 🜄 🜄

Weekly Tally & Notes

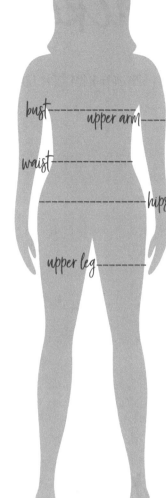

bust
upper arm
waist
hips
upper leg

Body Measurements:

BUST _____
UPPER ARM _____
WAIST _____
HIPS _____
UPPER LEG _____

Weekly Weight Tracker

CURRENT WEIGHT _____
GOAL WEIGHT _____

STRUGGLES

VICTORIES

Notes:

Never let a stumble in the road be the end of the journey.

Daily Fasting Tracker

	1AM	2AM	3AM	4AM	5AM	6AM	7AM	8AM	9AM	10AM	11AM	12PM	1PM	2PM	3PM	4PM	5PM	6PM	7PM	8PM	9PM	10PM	11PM	12AM
Monday	○	○	○	○	○	○	○	○	○	○	○	○	○	○	○	○	○	○	○	○	○	○	○	○
Tuesday	○	○	○	○	○	○	○	○	○	○	○	○	○	○	○	○	○	○	○	○	○	○	○	○
Wednesday	○	○	○	○	○	○	○	○	○	○	○	○	○	○	○	○	○	○	○	○	○	○	○	○
Thursday	○	○	○	○	○	○	○	○	○	○	○	○	○	○	○	○	○	○	○	○	○	○	○	○
Friday	○	○	○	○	○	○	○	○	○	○	○	○	○	○	○	○	○	○	○	○	○	○	○	○
Saturday	○	○	○	○	○	○	○	○	○	○	○	○	○	○	○	○	○	○	○	○	○	○	○	○
Sunday	○	○	○	○	○	○	○	○	○	○	○	○	○	○	○	○	○	○	○	○	○	○	○	○

Mood

MON
TUE
WED
THU
FRI
SAT
SUN

Daily Water Log

MON
TUES
WED
THU
FRI
SAT
SUN

Weekly Tally & Notes

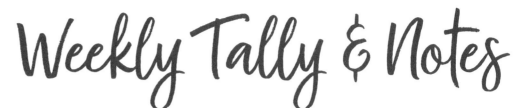

Body Measurements:

BUST _____
UPPER ARM _____
WAIST _____
HIPS _____
UPPER LEG _____

Weekly Weight Tracker

CURRENT WEIGHT _____
GOAL WEIGHT _____

STRUGGLES
VICTORIES

bust
upper arm
waist
hips
upper leg

Notes:

The process might be slow, but quitting won't speed it up.

Daily Fasting Tracker

	1AM	2AM	3AM	4AM	5AM	6AM	7AM	8AM	9AM	10AM	11AM	12PM	1PM	2PM	3PM	4PM	5PM	6PM	7PM	8PM	9PM	10PM	11PM	12AM
Monday	○	○	○	○	○	○	○	○	○	○	○	○	○	○	○	○	○	○	○	○	○	○	○	○
Tuesday	○	○	○	○	○	○	○	○	○	○	○	○	○	○	○	○	○	○	○	○	○	○	○	○
Wednesday	○	○	○	○	○	○	○	○	○	○	○	○	○	○	○	○	○	○	○	○	○	○	○	○
Thursday	○	○	○	○	○	○	○	○	○	○	○	○	○	○	○	○	○	○	○	○	○	○	○	○
Friday	○	○	○	○	○	○	○	○	○	○	○	○	○	○	○	○	○	○	○	○	○	○	○	○
Saturday	○	○	○	○	○	○	○	○	○	○	○	○	○	○	○	○	○	○	○	○	○	○	○	○
Sunday	○	○	○	○	○	○	○	○	○	○	○	○	○	○	○	○	○	○	○	○	○	○	○	○

Mood

MON
TUE
WED
THU
FRI
SAT
SUN

Daily Water Log

MON	○ ○ ○ ○ ○ ○ ○ ○
TUES	○ ○ ○ ○ ○ ○ ○ ○
WED	○ ○ ○ ○ ○ ○ ○ ○
THU	○ ○ ○ ○ ○ ○ ○ ○
FRI	○ ○ ○ ○ ○ ○ ○ ○
SAT	○ ○ ○ ○ ○ ○ ○ ○
SUN	○ ○ ○ ○ ○ ○ ○ ○

Weekly Tally & Notes

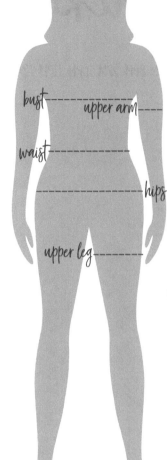

bust ----------
upper arm ----
waist ----------
hips ----
upper leg ----------

Body Measurements:

BUST _____
UPPER ARM _____
WAIST _____
HIPS _____
UPPER LEG _____

Weekly Weight Tracker

CURRENT WEIGHT _____
GOAL WEIGHT _____

STRUGGLES
VICTORIES

Notes:

Believe in the person you want to become.

Daily Fasting Tracker

	1AM	2AM	3AM	4AM	5AM	6AM	7AM	8AM	9AM	10AM	11AM	12PM	1PM	2PM	3PM	4PM	5PM	6PM	7PM	8PM	9PM	10PM	11PM	12AM
Monday	○	○	○	○	○	○	○	○	○	○	○	○	○	○	○	○	○	○	○	○	○	○	○	○
Tuesday	○	○	○	○	○	○	○	○	○	○	○	○	○	○	○	○	○	○	○	○	○	○	○	○
Wednesday	○	○	○	○	○	○	○	○	○	○	○	○	○	○	○	○	○	○	○	○	○	○	○	○
Thursday	○	○	○	○	○	○	○	○	○	○	○	○	○	○	○	○	○	○	○	○	○	○	○	○
Friday	○	○	○	○	○	○	○	○	○	○	○	○	○	○	○	○	○	○	○	○	○	○	○	○
Saturday	○	○	○	○	○	○	○	○	○	○	○	○	○	○	○	○	○	○	○	○	○	○	○	○
Sunday	○	○	○	○	○	○	○	○	○	○	○	○	○	○	○	○	○	○	○	○	○	○	○	○

Mood

MON
TUE
WED
THU
FRI
SAT
SUN

Daily Water Log

MON	◇ ◇ ◇ ◇ ◇ ◇ ◇ ◇
TUES	◇ ◇ ◇ ◇ ◇ ◇ ◇ ◇
WED	◇ ◇ ◇ ◇ ◇ ◇ ◇ ◇
THU	◇ ◇ ◇ ◇ ◇ ◇ ◇ ◇
FRI	◇ ◇ ◇ ◇ ◇ ◇ ◇ ◇
SAT	◇ ◇ ◇ ◇ ◇ ◇ ◇ ◇
SUN	◇ ◇ ◇ ◇ ◇ ◇ ◇ ◇

Weekly Tally & Notes

bust
upper arm
waist
hips
upper leg

Body Measurements:

BUST _____
UPPER ARM _____
WAIST _____
HIPS _____
UPPER LEG _____

Weekly Weight Tracker

CURRENT WEIGHT _____
GOAL WEIGHT _____

STRUGGLES
VICTORIES

Notes:

No grit, no pearl.

Daily Fasting Tracker

	1AM	2AM	3AM	4AM	5AM	6AM	7AM	8AM	9AM	10AM	11AM	12PM	1PM	2PM	3PM	4PM	5PM	6PM	7PM	8PM	9PM	10PM	11PM	12AM
Monday	○	○	○	○	○	○	○	○	○	○	○	○	○	○	○	○	○	○	○	○	○	○	○	○
Tuesday	○	○	○	○	○	○	○	○	○	○	○	○	○	○	○	○	○	○	○	○	○	○	○	○
Wednesday	○	○	○	○	○	○	○	○	○	○	○	○	○	○	○	○	○	○	○	○	○	○	○	○
Thursday	○	○	○	○	○	○	○	○	○	○	○	○	○	○	○	○	○	○	○	○	○	○	○	○
Friday	○	○	○	○	○	○	○	○	○	○	○	○	○	○	○	○	○	○	○	○	○	○	○	○
Saturday	○	○	○	○	○	○	○	○	○	○	○	○	○	○	○	○	○	○	○	○	○	○	○	○
Sunday	○	○	○	○	○	○	○	○	○	○	○	○	○	○	○	○	○	○	○	○	○	○	○	○

Mood

MON
TUE
WED
THU
FRI
SAT
SUN

Daily Water Log

MON	💧 💧 💧 💧 💧 💧 💧 💧
TUES	💧 💧 💧 💧 💧 💧 💧 💧
WED	💧 💧 💧 💧 💧 💧 💧 💧
THU	💧 💧 💧 💧 💧 💧 💧 💧
FRI	💧 💧 💧 💧 💧 💧 💧 💧
SAT	💧 💧 💧 💧 💧 💧 💧 💧
SUN	💧 💧 💧 💧 💧 💧 💧 💧

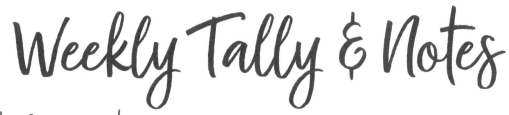

Weekly Tally & Notes

Body Measurements:

BUST	_____
UPPER ARM	_____
WAIST	_____
HIPS	_____
UPPER LEG	_____

Weekly Weight Tracker

CURRENT WEIGHT	_____
GOAL WEIGHT	_____

bust

upper arm

waist

hips

upper leg

STRUGGLES

VICTORIES

Notes:

Believe you can and you're halfway there.

Daily Fasting Tracker

	1AM	2AM	3AM	4AM	5AM	6AM	7AM	8AM	9AM	10AM	11AM	12PM	1PM	2PM	3PM	4PM	5PM	6PM	7PM	8PM	9PM	10PM	11PM	12AM
Monday	○	○	○	○	○	○	○	○	○	○	○	○	○	○	○	○	○	○	○	○	○	○	○	○
Tuesday	○	○	○	○	○	○	○	○	○	○	○	○	○	○	○	○	○	○	○	○	○	○	○	○
Wednesday	○	○	○	○	○	○	○	○	○	○	○	○	○	○	○	○	○	○	○	○	○	○	○	○
Thursday	○	○	○	○	○	○	○	○	○	○	○	○	○	○	○	○	○	○	○	○	○	○	○	○
Friday	○	○	○	○	○	○	○	○	○	○	○	○	○	○	○	○	○	○	○	○	○	○	○	○
Saturday	○	○	○	○	○	○	○	○	○	○	○	○	○	○	○	○	○	○	○	○	○	○	○	○
Sunday	○	○	○	○	○	○	○	○	○	○	○	○	○	○	○	○	○	○	○	○	○	○	○	○

Mood

MON
TUE
WED
THU
FRI
SAT
SUN

Daily Water Log

MON
TUES
WED
THU
FRI
SAT
SUN

Weekly Tally & Notes

Body Measurements:

BUST _____
UPPER ARM _____
WAIST _____
HIPS _____
UPPER LEG _____

Weekly Weight Tracker

CURRENT WEIGHT _____
GOAL WEIGHT _____

STRUGGLES
VICTORIES

bust
upper arm
waist
hips
upper leg

Notes:

Love yourself.

Daily Fasting Tracker

	1AM	2AM	3AM	4AM	5AM	6AM	7AM	8AM	9AM	10AM	11AM	12PM	1PM	2PM	3PM	4PM	5PM	6PM	7PM	8PM	9PM	10PM	11PM	12AM
Monday	○	○	○	○	○	○	○	○	○	○	○	○	○	○	○	○	○	○	○	○	○	○	○	○
Tuesday	○	○	○	○	○	○	○	○	○	○	○	○	○	○	○	○	○	○	○	○	○	○	○	○
Wednesday	○	○	○	○	○	○	○	○	○	○	○	○	○	○	○	○	○	○	○	○	○	○	○	○
Thursday	○	○	○	○	○	○	○	○	○	○	○	○	○	○	○	○	○	○	○	○	○	○	○	○
Friday	○	○	○	○	○	○	○	○	○	○	○	○	○	○	○	○	○	○	○	○	○	○	○	○
Saturday	○	○	○	○	○	○	○	○	○	○	○	○	○	○	○	○	○	○	○	○	○	○	○	○
Sunday	○	○	○	○	○	○	○	○	○	○	○	○	○	○	○	○	○	○	○	○	○	○	○	○

Mood

MON
TUE
WED
THU
FRI
SAT
SUN

Daily Water Log

MON	🜄 🜄 🜄 🜄 🜄 🜄 🜄 🜄
TUES	🜄 🜄 🜄 🜄 🜄 🜄 🜄 🜄
WED	🜄 🜄 🜄 🜄 🜄 🜄 🜄 🜄
THU	🜄 🜄 🜄 🜄 🜄 🜄 🜄 🜄
FRI	🜄 🜄 🜄 🜄 🜄 🜄 🜄 🜄
SAT	🜄 🜄 🜄 🜄 🜄 🜄 🜄 🜄
SUN	🜄 🜄 🜄 🜄 🜄 🜄 🜄 🜄

Weekly Tally & Notes

bust
upper arm
waist
hips
upper leg

Body Measurements:

BUST   _____
UPPER ARM   _____
WAIST   _____
HIPS   _____
UPPER LEG   _____

Weekly Weight Tracker

CURRENT WEIGHT   _____
GOAL WEIGHT   _____

STRUGGLES

VICTORIES

Notes:

No pressure, no diamonds.

Daily Fasting Tracker

	1AM	2AM	3AM	4AM	5AM	6AM	7AM	8AM	9AM	10AM	11AM	12PM	1PM	2PM	3PM	4PM	5PM	6PM	7PM	8PM	9PM	10PM	11PM	12AM
Monday	○	○	○	○	○	○	○	○	○	○	○	○	○	○	○	○	○	○	○	○	○	○	○	○
Tuesday	○	○	○	○	○	○	○	○	○	○	○	○	○	○	○	○	○	○	○	○	○	○	○	○
Wednesday	○	○	○	○	○	○	○	○	○	○	○	○	○	○	○	○	○	○	○	○	○	○	○	○
Thursday	○	○	○	○	○	○	○	○	○	○	○	○	○	○	○	○	○	○	○	○	○	○	○	○
Friday	○	○	○	○	○	○	○	○	○	○	○	○	○	○	○	○	○	○	○	○	○	○	○	○
Saturday	○	○	○	○	○	○	○	○	○	○	○	○	○	○	○	○	○	○	○	○	○	○	○	○
Sunday	○	○	○	○	○	○	○	○	○	○	○	○	○	○	○	○	○	○	○	○	○	○	○	○

Mood

MON
TUE
WED
THU
FRI
SAT
SUN

Daily Water Log

MON	◊ ◊ ◊ ◊ ◊ ◊ ◊ ◊
TUES	◊ ◊ ◊ ◊ ◊ ◊ ◊ ◊
WED	◊ ◊ ◊ ◊ ◊ ◊ ◊ ◊
THU	◊ ◊ ◊ ◊ ◊ ◊ ◊ ◊
FRI	◊ ◊ ◊ ◊ ◊ ◊ ◊ ◊
SAT	◊ ◊ ◊ ◊ ◊ ◊ ◊ ◊
SUN	◊ ◊ ◊ ◊ ◊ ◊ ◊ ◊

Weekly Tally & Notes

Body Measurements:

bust

upper arm

waist

hips

upper leg

BUST _____
UPPER ARM _____
WAIST _____
HIPS _____
UPPER LEG _____

Weekly Weight Tracker

CURRENT WEIGHT _____
GOAL WEIGHT _____

STRUGGLES

VICTORIES

Notes:

You can.

Daily Fasting Tracker

	1AM	2AM	3AM	4AM	5AM	6AM	7AM	8AM	9AM	10AM	11AM	12PM	1PM	2PM	3PM	4PM	5PM	6PM	7PM	8PM	9PM	10PM	11PM	12AM
Monday	○	○	○	○	○	○	○	○	○	○	○	○	○	○	○	○	○	○	○	○	○	○	○	○
Tuesday	○	○	○	○	○	○	○	○	○	○	○	○	○	○	○	○	○	○	○	○	○	○	○	○
Wednesday	○	○	○	○	○	○	○	○	○	○	○	○	○	○	○	○	○	○	○	○	○	○	○	○
Thursday	○	○	○	○	○	○	○	○	○	○	○	○	○	○	○	○	○	○	○	○	○	○	○	○
Friday	○	○	○	○	○	○	○	○	○	○	○	○	○	○	○	○	○	○	○	○	○	○	○	○
Saturday	○	○	○	○	○	○	○	○	○	○	○	○	○	○	○	○	○	○	○	○	○	○	○	○
Sunday	○	○	○	○	○	○	○	○	○	○	○	○	○	○	○	○	○	○	○	○	○	○	○	○

Mood

MON
TUE
WED
THU
FRI
SAT
SUN

Daily Water Log

MON
TUES
WED
THU
FRI
SAT
SUN

Weekly Tally & Notes

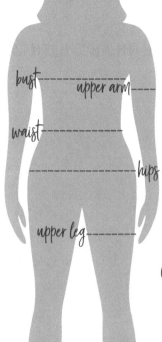

bust
upper arm
waist
hips
upper leg

Body Measurements:

BUST _____
UPPER ARM _____
WAIST _____
HIPS _____
UPPER LEG _____

Weekly Weight Tracker

CURRENT WEIGHT _____
GOAL WEIGHT _____

STRUGGLES

VICTORIES

Notes:

Don't decrease the goal, increase the effort.

Daily Fasting Tracker

	1AM	2AM	3AM	4AM	5AM	6AM	7AM	8AM	9AM	10AM	11AM	12PM	1PM	2PM	3PM	4PM	5PM	6PM	7PM	8PM	9PM	10PM	11PM	12AM
Monday	○	○	○	○	○	○	○	○	○	○	○	○	○	○	○	○	○	○	○	○	○	○	○	○
Tuesday	○	○	○	○	○	○	○	○	○	○	○	○	○	○	○	○	○	○	○	○	○	○	○	○
Wednesday	○	○	○	○	○	○	○	○	○	○	○	○	○	○	○	○	○	○	○	○	○	○	○	○
Thursday	○	○	○	○	○	○	○	○	○	○	○	○	○	○	○	○	○	○	○	○	○	○	○	○
Friday	○	○	○	○	○	○	○	○	○	○	○	○	○	○	○	○	○	○	○	○	○	○	○	○
Saturday	○	○	○	○	○	○	○	○	○	○	○	○	○	○	○	○	○	○	○	○	○	○	○	○
Sunday	○	○	○	○	○	○	○	○	○	○	○	○	○	○	○	○	○	○	○	○	○	○	○	○

Mood

MON
TUE
WED
THU
FRI
SAT
SUN

Daily Water Log

MON	🜄 🜄 🜄 🜄 🜄 🜄 🜄 🜄
TUES	🜄 🜄 🜄 🜄 🜄 🜄 🜄 🜄
WED	🜄 🜄 🜄 🜄 🜄 🜄 🜄 🜄
THU	🜄 🜄 🜄 🜄 🜄 🜄 🜄 🜄
FRI	🜄 🜄 🜄 🜄 🜄 🜄 🜄 🜄
SAT	🜄 🜄 🜄 🜄 🜄 🜄 🜄 🜄
SUN	🜄 🜄 🜄 🜄 🜄 🜄 🜄 🜄

Weekly Tally & Notes

bust
upper arm
waist
hips
upper leg

Body Measurements:

BUST _____
UPPER ARM _____
WAIST _____
HIPS _____
UPPER LEG _____

Weekly Weight Tracker

CURRENT WEIGHT _____
GOAL WEIGHT _____

STRUGGLES

VICTORIES

Notes:

If not now... Then when?

Daily Fasting Tracker

	1AM	2AM	3AM	4AM	5AM	6AM	7AM	8AM	9AM	10AM	11AM	12PM	1PM	2PM	3PM	4PM	5PM	6PM	7PM	8PM	9PM	10PM	11PM	12AM
Monday	○	○	○	○	○	○	○	○	○	○	○	○	○	○	○	○	○	○	○	○	○	○	○	○
Tuesday	○	○	○	○	○	○	○	○	○	○	○	○	○	○	○	○	○	○	○	○	○	○	○	○
Wednesday	○	○	○	○	○	○	○	○	○	○	○	○	○	○	○	○	○	○	○	○	○	○	○	○
Thursday	○	○	○	○	○	○	○	○	○	○	○	○	○	○	○	○	○	○	○	○	○	○	○	○
Friday	○	○	○	○	○	○	○	○	○	○	○	○	○	○	○	○	○	○	○	○	○	○	○	○
Saturday	○	○	○	○	○	○	○	○	○	○	○	○	○	○	○	○	○	○	○	○	○	○	○	○
Sunday	○	○	○	○	○	○	○	○	○	○	○	○	○	○	○	○	○	○	○	○	○	○	○	○

Mood

MON
TUE
WED
THU
FRI
SAT
SUN

Daily Water Log

MON
TUES
WED
THU
FRI
SAT
SUN

Weekly Tally & Notes

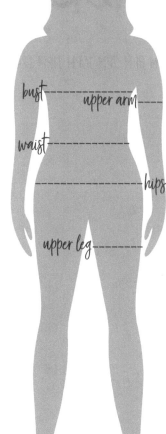

bust
upper arm
waist
hips
upper leg

Body Measurements:

BUST _____
UPPER ARM _____
WAIST _____
HIPS _____
UPPER LEG _____

Weekly Weight Tracker

CURRENT WEIGHT _____
GOAL WEIGHT _____

STRUGGLES

VICTORIES

Notes:

It always seems impossible until it's done.

Daily Fasting Tracker

	1AM	2AM	3AM	4AM	5AM	6AM	7AM	8AM	9AM	10AM	11AM	12PM	1PM	2PM	3PM	4PM	5PM	6PM	7PM	8PM	9PM	10PM	11PM	12AM
Monday	○	○	○	○	○	○	○	○	○	○	○	○	○	○	○	○	○	○	○	○	○	○	○	○
Tuesday	○	○	○	○	○	○	○	○	○	○	○	○	○	○	○	○	○	○	○	○	○	○	○	○
Wednesday	○	○	○	○	○	○	○	○	○	○	○	○	○	○	○	○	○	○	○	○	○	○	○	○
Thursday	○	○	○	○	○	○	○	○	○	○	○	○	○	○	○	○	○	○	○	○	○	○	○	○
Friday	○	○	○	○	○	○	○	○	○	○	○	○	○	○	○	○	○	○	○	○	○	○	○	○
Saturday	○	○	○	○	○	○	○	○	○	○	○	○	○	○	○	○	○	○	○	○	○	○	○	○
Sunday	○	○	○	○	○	○	○	○	○	○	○	○	○	○	○	○	○	○	○	○	○	○	○	○

Mood

MON
TUE
WED
THU
FRI
SAT
SUN

Daily Water Log

MON
TUES
WED
THU
FRI
SAT
SUN

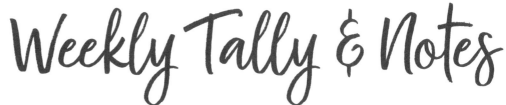

Weekly Tally & Notes

Body Measurements:

BUST _____
UPPER ARM _____
WAIST _____
HIPS _____
UPPER LEG _____

Weekly Weight Tracker

CURRENT WEIGHT _____
GOAL WEIGHT _____

bust
upper arm
waist
hips
upper leg

STRUGGLES

VICTORIES

Notes:

Your goals don't care how you feel.

Daily Fasting Tracker

	1AM	2AM	3AM	4AM	5AM	6AM	7AM	8AM	9AM	10AM	11AM	12PM	1PM	2PM	3PM	4PM	5PM	6PM	7PM	8PM	9PM	10PM	11PM	12AM
Monday	○	○	○	○	○	○	○	○	○	○	○	○	○	○	○	○	○	○	○	○	○	○	○	○
Tuesday	○	○	○	○	○	○	○	○	○	○	○	○	○	○	○	○	○	○	○	○	○	○	○	○
Wednesday	○	○	○	○	○	○	○	○	○	○	○	○	○	○	○	○	○	○	○	○	○	○	○	○
Thursday	○	○	○	○	○	○	○	○	○	○	○	○	○	○	○	○	○	○	○	○	○	○	○	○
Friday	○	○	○	○	○	○	○	○	○	○	○	○	○	○	○	○	○	○	○	○	○	○	○	○
Saturday	○	○	○	○	○	○	○	○	○	○	○	○	○	○	○	○	○	○	○	○	○	○	○	○
Sunday	○	○	○	○	○	○	○	○	○	○	○	○	○	○	○	○	○	○	○	○	○	○	○	○

Mood

MON
TUE
WED
THU
FRI
SAT
SUN

Daily Water Log

MON	🜄 🜄 🜄 🜄 🜄 🜄 🜄 🜄
TUES	🜄 🜄 🜄 🜄 🜄 🜄 🜄 🜄
WED	🜄 🜄 🜄 🜄 🜄 🜄 🜄 🜄
THU	🜄 🜄 🜄 🜄 🜄 🜄 🜄 🜄
FRI	🜄 🜄 🜄 🜄 🜄 🜄 🜄 🜄
SAT	🜄 🜄 🜄 🜄 🜄 🜄 🜄 🜄
SUN	🜄 🜄 🜄 🜄 🜄 🜄 🜄 🜄

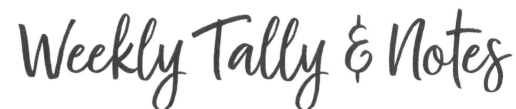

Weekly Tally & Notes

bust———————
upper arm————
waist———————
————————hips
upper leg————

Body Measurements:

BUST _____
UPPER ARM _____
WAIST _____
HIPS _____
UPPER LEG _____

Weekly Weight Tracker

CURRENT WEIGHT _____
GOAL WEIGHT _____

STRUGGLES

VICTORIES

Notes:

Success is an inside job.

Daily Fasting Tracker

	1AM	2AM	3AM	4AM	5AM	6AM	7AM	8AM	9AM	10AM	11AM	12PM	1PM	2PM	3PM	4PM	5PM	6PM	7PM	8PM	9PM	10PM	11PM	12AM
Monday	○	○	○	○	○	○	○	○	○	○	○	○	○	○	○	○	○	○	○	○	○	○	○	○
Tuesday	○	○	○	○	○	○	○	○	○	○	○	○	○	○	○	○	○	○	○	○	○	○	○	○
Wednesday	○	○	○	○	○	○	○	○	○	○	○	○	○	○	○	○	○	○	○	○	○	○	○	○
Thursday	○	○	○	○	○	○	○	○	○	○	○	○	○	○	○	○	○	○	○	○	○	○	○	○
Friday	○	○	○	○	○	○	○	○	○	○	○	○	○	○	○	○	○	○	○	○	○	○	○	○
Saturday	○	○	○	○	○	○	○	○	○	○	○	○	○	○	○	○	○	○	○	○	○	○	○	○
Sunday	○	○	○	○	○	○	○	○	○	○	○	○	○	○	○	○	○	○	○	○	○	○	○	○

Mood

MON
TUE
WED
THU
FRI
SAT
SUN

Daily Water Log

MON	〇 〇 〇 〇 〇 〇 〇 〇
TUES	〇 〇 〇 〇 〇 〇 〇 〇
WED	〇 〇 〇 〇 〇 〇 〇 〇
THU	〇 〇 〇 〇 〇 〇 〇
FRI	〇 〇 〇 〇 〇 〇 〇
SAT	〇 〇 〇 〇 〇 〇 〇
SUN	〇 〇 〇 〇 〇 〇 〇

Weekly Tally & Notes

Body Measurements:

BUST _____
UPPER ARM _____
WAIST _____
HIPS _____
UPPER LEG _____

Weekly Weight Tracker

CURRENT WEIGHT _____
GOAL WEIGHT _____

Notes:

bust
upper arm
waist
hips
upper leg

STRUGGLES

VICTORIES

Find a way, not an excuse.

Daily Fasting Tracker

	1AM	2AM	3AM	4AM	5AM	6AM	7AM	8AM	9AM	10AM	11AM	12PM	1PM	2PM	3PM	4PM	5PM	6PM	7PM	8PM	9PM	10PM	11PM	12AM
Monday	○	○	○	○	○	○	○	○	○	○	○	○	○	○	○	○	○	○	○	○	○	○	○	○
Tuesday	○	○	○	○	○	○	○	○	○	○	○	○	○	○	○	○	○	○	○	○	○	○	○	○
Wednesday	○	○	○	○	○	○	○	○	○	○	○	○	○	○	○	○	○	○	○	○	○	○	○	○
Thursday	○	○	○	○	○	○	○	○	○	○	○	○	○	○	○	○	○	○	○	○	○	○	○	○
Friday	○	○	○	○	○	○	○	○	○	○	○	○	○	○	○	○	○	○	○	○	○	○	○	○
Saturday	○	○	○	○	○	○	○	○	○	○	○	○	○	○	○	○	○	○	○	○	○	○	○	○
Sunday	○	○	○	○	○	○	○	○	○	○	○	○	○	○	○	○	○	○	○	○	○	○	○	○

Mood

MON
TUE
WED
THU
FRI
SAT
SUN

Daily Water Log

MON
TUES
WED
THU
FRI
SAT
SUN

Weekly Tally & Notes

bust ----------
upper arm ----
waist ----------
hips
upper leg ----------

Body Measurements:

BUST _____
UPPER ARM _____
WAIST _____
HIPS _____
UPPER LEG _____

Weekly Weight Tracker

CURRENT WEIGHT _____
GOAL WEIGHT _____

STRUGGLES

VICTORIES

Notes:

Be the change you want to see.

Daily Fasting Tracker

	1AM	2AM	3AM	4AM	5AM	6AM	7AM	8AM	9AM	10AM	11AM	12PM	1PM	2PM	3PM	4PM	5PM	6PM	7PM	8PM	9PM	10PM	11PM	12AM
Monday	○	○	○	○	○	○	○	○	○	○	○	○	○	○	○	○	○	○	○	○	○	○	○	○
Tuesday	○	○	○	○	○	○	○	○	○	○	○	○	○	○	○	○	○	○	○	○	○	○	○	○
Wednesday	○	○	○	○	○	○	○	○	○	○	○	○	○	○	○	○	○	○	○	○	○	○	○	○
Thursday	○	○	○	○	○	○	○	○	○	○	○	○	○	○	○	○	○	○	○	○	○	○	○	○
Friday	○	○	○	○	○	○	○	○	○	○	○	○	○	○	○	○	○	○	○	○	○	○	○	○
Saturday	○	○	○	○	○	○	○	○	○	○	○	○	○	○	○	○	○	○	○	○	○	○	○	○
Sunday	○	○	○	○	○	○	○	○	○	○	○	○	○	○	○	○	○	○	○	○	○	○	○	○

Mood

MON
TUE
WED
THU
FRI
SAT
SUN

Daily Water Log

MON	○ ○ ○ ○ ○ ○ ○ ○
TUES	○ ○ ○ ○ ○ ○ ○ ○
WED	○ ○ ○ ○ ○ ○ ○ ○
THU	○ ○ ○ ○ ○ ○ ○ ○
FRI	○ ○ ○ ○ ○ ○ ○ ○
SAT	○ ○ ○ ○ ○ ○ ○ ○
SUN	○ ○ ○ ○ ○ ○ ○ ○

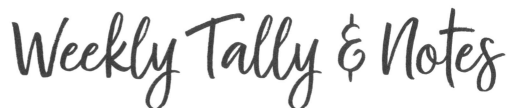

Weekly Tally & Notes

body measurements labels on figure: bust, upper arm, waist, hips, upper leg

Body Measurements:

BUST _____
UPPER ARM _____
WAIST _____
HIPS _____
UPPER LEG _____

Weekly Weight Tracker

CURRENT WEIGHT _____
GOAL WEIGHT _____

STRUGGLES

VICTORIES

Notes:

Work hard and make it happen.

Daily Fasting Tracker

	1AM	2AM	3AM	4AM	5AM	6AM	7AM	8AM	9AM	10AM	11AM	12PM	1PM	2PM	3PM	4PM	5PM	6PM	7PM	8PM	9PM	10PM	11PM	12AM
Monday	○	○	○	○	○	○	○	○	○	○	○	○	○	○	○	○	○	○	○	○	○	○	○	○
Tuesday	○	○	○	○	○	○	○	○	○	○	○	○	○	○	○	○	○	○	○	○	○	○	○	○
Wednesday	○	○	○	○	○	○	○	○	○	○	○	○	○	○	○	○	○	○	○	○	○	○	○	○
Thursday	○	○	○	○	○	○	○	○	○	○	○	○	○	○	○	○	○	○	○	○	○	○	○	○
Friday	○	○	○	○	○	○	○	○	○	○	○	○	○	○	○	○	○	○	○	○	○	○	○	○
Saturday	○	○	○	○	○	○	○	○	○	○	○	○	○	○	○	○	○	○	○	○	○	○	○	○
Sunday	○	○	○	○	○	○	○	○	○	○	○	○	○	○	○	○	○	○	○	○	○	○	○	○

Mood

MON
TUE
WED
THU
FRI
SAT
SUN

Daily Water Log

MON	○ ○ ○ ○ ○ ○ ○ ○
TUES	○ ○ ○ ○ ○ ○ ○ ○
WED	○ ○ ○ ○ ○ ○ ○ ○
THU	○ ○ ○ ○ ○ ○ ○ ○
FRI	○ ○ ○ ○ ○ ○ ○ ○
SAT	○ ○ ○ ○ ○ ○ ○ ○
SUN	○ ○ ○ ○ ○ ○ ○ ○

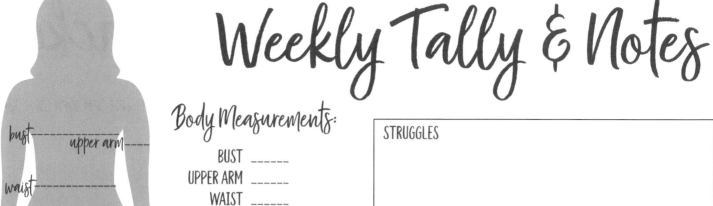

Weekly Tally & Notes

Body Measurements:

BUST	_____
UPPER ARM	_____
WAIST	_____
HIPS	_____
UPPER LEG	_____

Weekly Weight Tracker

CURRENT WEIGHT	_____
GOAL WEIGHT	_____

bust

upper arm

waist

hips

upper leg

STRUGGLES

VICTORIES

Notes:

Be the best version of you.

Daily Fasting Tracker

	1AM	2AM	3AM	4AM	5AM	6AM	7AM	8AM	9AM	10AM	11AM	12PM	1PM	2PM	3PM	4PM	5PM	6PM	7PM	8PM	9PM	10PM	11PM	12AM
Monday	○	○	○	○	○	○	○	○	○	○	○	○	○	○	○	○	○	○	○	○	○	○	○	○
Tuesday	○	○	○	○	○	○	○	○	○	○	○	○	○	○	○	○	○	○	○	○	○	○	○	○
Wednesday	○	○	○	○	○	○	○	○	○	○	○	○	○	○	○	○	○	○	○	○	○	○	○	○
Thursday	○	○	○	○	○	○	○	○	○	○	○	○	○	○	○	○	○	○	○	○	○	○	○	○
Friday	○	○	○	○	○	○	○	○	○	○	○	○	○	○	○	○	○	○	○	○	○	○	○	○
Saturday	○	○	○	○	○	○	○	○	○	○	○	○	○	○	○	○	○	○	○	○	○	○	○	○
Sunday	○	○	○	○	○	○	○	○	○	○	○	○	○	○	○	○	○	○	○	○	○	○	○	○

Mood

MON
TUE
WED
THU
FRI
SAT
SUN

Daily Water Log

MON	◊ ◊ ◊ ◊ ◊ ◊ ◊ ◊
TUES	◊ ◊ ◊ ◊ ◊ ◊ ◊ ◊
WED	◊ ◊ ◊ ◊ ◊ ◊ ◊ ◊
THU	◊ ◊ ◊ ◊ ◊ ◊ ◊ ◊
FRI	◊ ◊ ◊ ◊ ◊ ◊ ◊ ◊
SAT	◊ ◊ ◊ ◊ ◊ ◊ ◊ ◊
SUN	◊ ◊ ◊ ◊ ◊ ◊ ◊ ◊

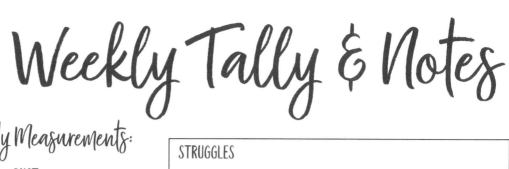

Weekly Tally & Notes

Body Measurements:

BUST _____
UPPER ARM _____
WAIST _____
HIPS _____
UPPER LEG _____

bust
upper arm
waist
hips
upper leg

Weekly Weight Tracker

CURRENT WEIGHT _____
GOAL WEIGHT _____

STRUGGLES

VICTORIES

Notes:

Your attitude determines your direction.

Daily Fasting Tracker

	1AM	2AM	3AM	4AM	5AM	6AM	7AM	8AM	9AM	10AM	11AM	12PM	1PM	2PM	3PM	4PM	5PM	6PM	7PM	8PM	9PM	10PM	11PM	12AM
Monday	○	○	○	○	○	○	○	○	○	○	○	○	○	○	○	○	○	○	○	○	○	○	○	○
Tuesday	○	○	○	○	○	○	○	○	○	○	○	○	○	○	○	○	○	○	○	○	○	○	○	○
Wednesday	○	○	○	○	○	○	○	○	○	○	○	○	○	○	○	○	○	○	○	○	○	○	○	○
Thursday	○	○	○	○	○	○	○	○	○	○	○	○	○	○	○	○	○	○	○	○	○	○	○	○
Friday	○	○	○	○	○	○	○	○	○	○	○	○	○	○	○	○	○	○	○	○	○	○	○	○
Saturday	○	○	○	○	○	○	○	○	○	○	○	○	○	○	○	○	○	○	○	○	○	○	○	○
Sunday	○	○	○	○	○	○	○	○	○	○	○	○	○	○	○	○	○	○	○	○	○	○	○	○

Mood

MON
TUE
WED
THU
FRI
SAT
SUN

Daily Water Log

MON	◇ ◇ ◇ ◇ ◇ ◇ ◇ ◇
TUES	◇ ◇ ◇ ◇ ◇ ◇ ◇ ◇
WED	◇ ◇ ◇ ◇ ◇ ◇ ◇ ◇
THU	◇ ◇ ◇ ◇ ◇ ◇ ◇ ◇
FRI	◇ ◇ ◇ ◇ ◇ ◇ ◇ ◇
SAT	◇ ◇ ◇ ◇ ◇ ◇ ◇ ◇
SUN	◇ ◇ ◇ ◇ ◇ ◇ ◇ ◇

Weekly Tally & Notes

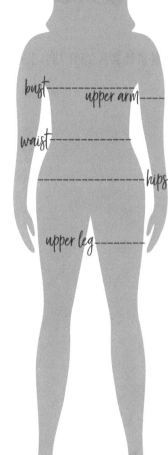

bust
upper arm
waist
hips
upper leg

Body Measurements:

BUST _____
UPPER ARM _____
WAIST _____
HIPS _____
UPPER LEG _____

Weekly Weight Tracker

CURRENT WEIGHT _____
GOAL WEIGHT _____

STRUGGLES

VICTORIES

Notes:

Amazing things happen when you try.

Daily Fasting Tracker

	1AM	2AM	3AM	4AM	5AM	6AM	7AM	8AM	9AM	10AM	11AM	12PM	1PM	2PM	3PM	4PM	5PM	6PM	7PM	8PM	9PM	10PM	11PM	12AM
Monday	○	○	○	○	○	○	○	○	○	○	○	○	○	○	○	○	○	○	○	○	○	○	○	○
Tuesday	○	○	○	○	○	○	○	○	○	○	○	○	○	○	○	○	○	○	○	○	○	○	○	○
Wednesday	○	○	○	○	○	○	○	○	○	○	○	○	○	○	○	○	○	○	○	○	○	○	○	○
Thursday	○	○	○	○	○	○	○	○	○	○	○	○	○	○	○	○	○	○	○	○	○	○	○	○
Friday	○	○	○	○	○	○	○	○	○	○	○	○	○	○	○	○	○	○	○	○	○	○	○	○
Saturday	○	○	○	○	○	○	○	○	○	○	○	○	○	○	○	○	○	○	○	○	○	○	○	○
Sunday	○	○	○	○	○	○	○	○	○	○	○	○	○	○	○	○	○	○	○	○	○	○	○	○

Mood

MON
TUE
WED
THU
FRI
SAT
SUN

Daily Water Log

MON	◇ ◇ ◇ ◇ ◇ ◇ ◇ ◇
TUES	◇ ◇ ◇ ◇ ◇ ◇ ◇ ◇
WED	◇ ◇ ◇ ◇ ◇ ◇ ◇
THU	◇ ◇ ◇ ◇ ◇ ◇ ◇ ◇
FRI	◇ ◇ ◇ ◇ ◇ ◇ ◇ ◇
SAT	◇ ◇ ◇ ◇ ◇ ◇ ◇
SUN	◇ ◇ ◇ ◇ ◇ ◇ ◇

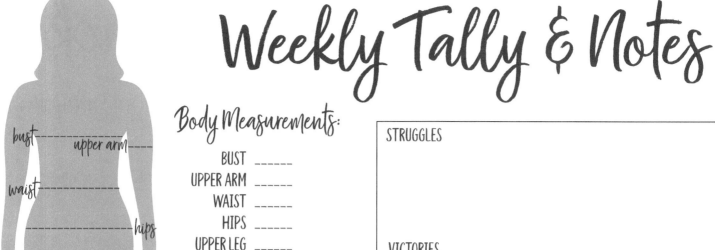

Weekly Tally & Notes

Body Measurements:

BUST _____
UPPER ARM _____
WAIST _____
HIPS _____
UPPER LEG _____

Weekly Weight Tracker

CURRENT WEIGHT _____
GOAL WEIGHT _____

bust
upper arm
waist
hips
upper leg

STRUGGLES

VICTORIES

Notes:

The only way you see results is if you stay consistent.

Daily Fasting Tracker

	1AM	2AM	3AM	4AM	5AM	6AM	7AM	8AM	9AM	10AM	11AM	12PM	1PM	2PM	3PM	4PM	5PM	6PM	7PM	8PM	9PM	10PM	11PM	12AM
Monday	○	○	○	○	○	○	○	○	○	○	○	○	○	○	○	○	○	○	○	○	○	○	○	○
Tuesday	○	○	○	○	○	○	○	○	○	○	○	○	○	○	○	○	○	○	○	○	○	○	○	○
Wednesday	○	○	○	○	○	○	○	○	○	○	○	○	○	○	○	○	○	○	○	○	○	○	○	○
Thursday	○	○	○	○	○	○	○	○	○	○	○	○	○	○	○	○	○	○	○	○	○	○	○	○
Friday	○	○	○	○	○	○	○	○	○	○	○	○	○	○	○	○	○	○	○	○	○	○	○	○
Saturday	○	○	○	○	○	○	○	○	○	○	○	○	○	○	○	○	○	○	○	○	○	○	○	○
Sunday	○	○	○	○	○	○	○	○	○	○	○	○	○	○	○	○	○	○	○	○	○	○	○	○

Mood

MON
TUE
WED
THU
FRI
SAT
SUN

Daily Water Log

MON
TUES
WED
THU
FRI
SAT
SUN

Weekly Tally & Notes

bust----------
upper arm-----
waist----------
----------hips
upper leg----------

Body Measurements:

BUST _____
UPPER ARM _____
WAIST _____
HIPS _____
UPPER LEG _____

Weekly Weight Tracker

CURRENT WEIGHT _____
GOAL WEIGHT _____

STRUGGLES

VICTORIES

Notes:

Flowers need time to bloom, so do you.

Daily Fasting Tracker

	1AM	2AM	3AM	4AM	5AM	6AM	7AM	8AM	9AM	10AM	11AM	12PM	1PM	2PM	3PM	4PM	5PM	6PM	7PM	8PM	9PM	10PM	11PM	12AM
Monday	○	○	○	○	○	○	○	○	○	○	○	○	○	○	○	○	○	○	○	○	○	○	○	○
Tuesday	○	○	○	○	○	○	○	○	○	○	○	○	○	○	○	○	○	○	○	○	○	○	○	○
Wednesday	○	○	○	○	○	○	○	○	○	○	○	○	○	○	○	○	○	○	○	○	○	○	○	○
Thursday	○	○	○	○	○	○	○	○	○	○	○	○	○	○	○	○	○	○	○	○	○	○	○	○
Friday	○	○	○	○	○	○	○	○	○	○	○	○	○	○	○	○	○	○	○	○	○	○	○	○
Saturday	○	○	○	○	○	○	○	○	○	○	○	○	○	○	○	○	○	○	○	○	○	○	○	○
Sunday	○	○	○	○	○	○	○	○	○	○	○	○	○	○	○	○	○	○	○	○	○	○	○	○

Mood

MON
TUE
WED
THU
FRI
SAT
SUN

Daily Water Log

MON								
TUES								
WED								
THU								
FRI								
SAT								
SUN								

Weekly Tally & Notes

bust
upper arm
waist
hips
upper leg

Body Measurements:

BUST _____
UPPER ARM _____
WAIST _____
HIPS _____
UPPER LEG _____

Weekly Weight Tracker

CURRENT WEIGHT _____
GOAL WEIGHT _____

STRUGGLES

VICTORIES

Notes:

Trust the process.

Daily Fasting Tracker

	1AM	2AM	3AM	4AM	5AM	6AM	7AM	8AM	9AM	10AM	11AM	12PM	1PM	2PM	3PM	4PM	5PM	6PM	7PM	8PM	9PM	10PM	11PM	12AM
Monday	○	○	○	○	○	○	○	○	○	○	○	○	○	○	○	○	○	○	○	○	○	○	○	○
Tuesday	○	○	○	○	○	○	○	○	○	○	○	○	○	○	○	○	○	○	○	○	○	○	○	○
Wednesday	○	○	○	○	○	○	○	○	○	○	○	○	○	○	○	○	○	○	○	○	○	○	○	○
Thursday	○	○	○	○	○	○	○	○	○	○	○	○	○	○	○	○	○	○	○	○	○	○	○	○
Friday	○	○	○	○	○	○	○	○	○	○	○	○	○	○	○	○	○	○	○	○	○	○	○	○
Saturday	○	○	○	○	○	○	○	○	○	○	○	○	○	○	○	○	○	○	○	○	○	○	○	○
Sunday	○	○	○	○	○	○	○	○	○	○	○	○	○	○	○	○	○	○	○	○	○	○	○	○

Mood

MON
TUE
WED
THU
FRI
SAT
SUN

Daily Water Log

MON	◊ ◊ ◊ ◊ ◊ ◊ ◊ ◊
TUES	◊ ◊ ◊ ◊ ◊ ◊ ◊
WED	◊ ◊ ◊ ◊ ◊ ◊ ◊
THU	◊ ◊ ◊ ◊ ◊ ◊ ◊ ◊
FRI	◊ ◊ ◊ ◊ ◊ ◊ ◊
SAT	◊ ◊ ◊ ◊ ◊ ◊ ◊
SUN	◊ ◊ ◊ ◊ ◊ ◊ ◊

Weekly Tally & Notes

labels on figure: bust, upper arm, waist, hips, upper leg

Body Measurements:

BUST _____
UPPER ARM _____
WAIST _____
HIPS _____
UPPER LEG _____

Weekly Weight Tracker

CURRENT WEIGHT _____
GOAL WEIGHT _____

STRUGGLES

VICTORIES

Notes:

Success = 20% strategy + 80% mindset

Daily Fasting Tracker

	1AM	2AM	3AM	4AM	5AM	6AM	7AM	8AM	9AM	10AM	11AM	12PM	1PM	2PM	3PM	4PM	5PM	6PM	7PM	8PM	9PM	10PM	11PM	12AM
Monday	○	○	○	○	○	○	○	○	○	○	○	○	○	○	○	○	○	○	○	○	○	○	○	○
Tuesday	○	○	○	○	○	○	○	○	○	○	○	○	○	○	○	○	○	○	○	○	○	○	○	○
Wednesday	○	○	○	○	○	○	○	○	○	○	○	○	○	○	○	○	○	○	○	○	○	○	○	○
Thursday	○	○	○	○	○	○	○	○	○	○	○	○	○	○	○	○	○	○	○	○	○	○	○	○
Friday	○	○	○	○	○	○	○	○	○	○	○	○	○	○	○	○	○	○	○	○	○	○	○	○
Saturday	○	○	○	○	○	○	○	○	○	○	○	○	○	○	○	○	○	○	○	○	○	○	○	○
Sunday	○	○	○	○	○	○	○	○	○	○	○	○	○	○	○	○	○	○	○	○	○	○	○	○

Mood

MON
TUE
WED
THU
FRI
SAT
SUN

Daily Water Log

MON
TUES
WED
THU
FRI
SAT
SUN

Weekly Tally & Notes

Body Measurements:

BUST _____
UPPER ARM _____
WAIST _____
HIPS _____
UPPER LEG _____

Weekly Weight Tracker

CURRENT WEIGHT _____
GOAL WEIGHT _____

bust
upper arm
waist
hips
upper leg

STRUGGLES

VICTORIES

Notes:

Good things take time.

Daily Fasting Tracker

	1AM	2AM	3AM	4AM	5AM	6AM	7AM	8AM	9AM	10AM	11AM	12PM	1PM	2PM	3PM	4PM	5PM	6PM	7PM	8PM	9PM	10PM	11PM	12AM
Monday	○	○	○	○	○	○	○	○	○	○	○	○	○	○	○	○	○	○	○	○	○	○	○	○
Tuesday	○	○	○	○	○	○	○	○	○	○	○	○	○	○	○	○	○	○	○	○	○	○	○	○
Wednesday	○	○	○	○	○	○	○	○	○	○	○	○	○	○	○	○	○	○	○	○	○	○	○	○
Thursday	○	○	○	○	○	○	○	○	○	○	○	○	○	○	○	○	○	○	○	○	○	○	○	○
Friday	○	○	○	○	○	○	○	○	○	○	○	○	○	○	○	○	○	○	○	○	○	○	○	○
Saturday	○	○	○	○	○	○	○	○	○	○	○	○	○	○	○	○	○	○	○	○	○	○	○	○
Sunday	○	○	○	○	○	○	○	○	○	○	○	○	○	○	○	○	○	○	○	○	○	○	○	○

Mood

MON

TUE

WED

THU

FRI

SAT

SUN

Daily Water Log

MON

TUES

WED

THU

FRI

SAT

SUN

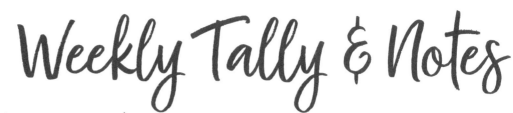

Weekly Tally & Notes

Body Measurements:

BUST _____
UPPER ARM _____
WAIST _____
HIPS _____
UPPER LEG _____

Weekly Weight Tracker

CURRENT WEIGHT _____
GOAL WEIGHT _____

bust
upper arm
waist
hips
upper leg

STRUGGLES

VICTORIES

Notes:

Make yourself a priority.

Daily Fasting Tracker

	1AM	2AM	3AM	4AM	5AM	6AM	7AM	8AM	9AM	10AM	11AM	12PM	1PM	2PM	3PM	4PM	5PM	6PM	7PM	8PM	9PM	10PM	11PM	12AM
Monday	○	○	○	○	○	○	○	○	○	○	○	○	○	○	○	○	○	○	○	○	○	○	○	○
Tuesday	○	○	○	○	○	○	○	○	○	○	○	○	○	○	○	○	○	○	○	○	○	○	○	○
Wednesday	○	○	○	○	○	○	○	○	○	○	○	○	○	○	○	○	○	○	○	○	○	○	○	○
Thursday	○	○	○	○	○	○	○	○	○	○	○	○	○	○	○	○	○	○	○	○	○	○	○	○
Friday	○	○	○	○	○	○	○	○	○	○	○	○	○	○	○	○	○	○	○	○	○	○	○	○
Saturday	○	○	○	○	○	○	○	○	○	○	○	○	○	○	○	○	○	○	○	○	○	○	○	○
Sunday	○	○	○	○	○	○	○	○	○	○	○	○	○	○	○	○	○	○	○	○	○	○	○	○

Mood

MON
TUE
WED
THU
FRI
SAT
SUN

Daily Water Log

MON	🜄 🜄 🜄 🜄 🜄 🜄 🜄 🜄
TUES	🜄 🜄 🜄 🜄 🜄 🜄 🜄 🜄
WED	🜄 🜄 🜄 🜄 🜄 🜄 🜄 🜄
THU	🜄 🜄 🜄 🜄 🜄 🜄 🜄 🜄
FRI	🜄 🜄 🜄 🜄 🜄 🜄 🜄 🜄
SAT	🜄 🜄 🜄 🜄 🜄 🜄 🜄 🜄
SUN	🜄 🜄 🜄 🜄 🜄 🜄 🜄 🜄

Weekly Tally & Notes

Body Measurements:

bust

upper arm

waist

hips

upper leg

BUST _____

UPPER ARM _____

WAIST _____

HIPS _____

UPPER LEG _____

Weekly Weight Tracker

CURRENT WEIGHT _____

GOAL WEIGHT _____

STRUGGLES

VICTORIES

Notes:

If you want it, work for it.

Daily Fasting Tracker

	1AM	2AM	3AM	4AM	5AM	6AM	7AM	8AM	9AM	10AM	11AM	12PM	1PM	2PM	3PM	4PM	5PM	6PM	7PM	8PM	9PM	10PM	11PM	12AM
Monday	○	○	○	○	○	○	○	○	○	○	○	○	○	○	○	○	○	○	○	○	○	○	○	○
Tuesday	○	○	○	○	○	○	○	○	○	○	○	○	○	○	○	○	○	○	○	○	○	○	○	○
Wednesday	○	○	○	○	○	○	○	○	○	○	○	○	○	○	○	○	○	○	○	○	○	○	○	○
Thursday	○	○	○	○	○	○	○	○	○	○	○	○	○	○	○	○	○	○	○	○	○	○	○	○
Friday	○	○	○	○	○	○	○	○	○	○	○	○	○	○	○	○	○	○	○	○	○	○	○	○
Saturday	○	○	○	○	○	○	○	○	○	○	○	○	○	○	○	○	○	○	○	○	○	○	○	○
Sunday	○	○	○	○	○	○	○	○	○	○	○	○	○	○	○	○	○	○	○	○	○	○	○	○

Mood

MON
TUE
WED
THU
FRI
SAT
SUN

Daily Water Log

MON	🜄 🜄 🜄 🜄 🜄 🜄 🜄 🜄
TUES	🜄 🜄 🜄 🜄 🜄 🜄 🜄 🜄
WED	🜄 🜄 🜄 🜄 🜄 🜄 🜄 🜄
THU	🜄 🜄 🜄 🜄 🜄 🜄 🜄 🜄
FRI	🜄 🜄 🜄 🜄 🜄 🜄 🜄 🜄
SAT	🜄 🜄 🜄 🜄 🜄 🜄 🜄 🜄
SUN	🜄 🜄 🜄 🜄 🜄 🜄 🜄 🜄

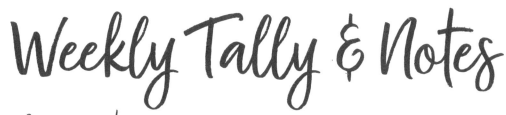

Weekly Tally & Notes

bust ------- upper arm ----
waist -----------------
------------- hips
upper leg ------------

Body Measurements:

BUST _____
UPPER ARM _____
WAIST _____
HIPS _____
UPPER LEG _____

Weekly Weight Tracker

CURRENT WEIGHT _____
GOAL WEIGHT _____

STRUGGLES

VICTORIES

Notes:

There is no change where there is no action.

Daily Fasting Tracker

	1AM	2AM	3AM	4AM	5AM	6AM	7AM	8AM	9AM	10AM	11AM	12PM	1PM	2PM	3PM	4PM	5PM	6PM	7PM	8PM	9PM	10PM	11PM	12AM
Monday	○	○	○	○	○	○	○	○	○	○	○	○	○	○	○	○	○	○	○	○	○	○	○	○
Tuesday	○	○	○	○	○	○	○	○	○	○	○	○	○	○	○	○	○	○	○	○	○	○	○	○
Wednesday	○	○	○	○	○	○	○	○	○	○	○	○	○	○	○	○	○	○	○	○	○	○	○	○
Thursday	○	○	○	○	○	○	○	○	○	○	○	○	○	○	○	○	○	○	○	○	○	○	○	○
Friday	○	○	○	○	○	○	○	○	○	○	○	○	○	○	○	○	○	○	○	○	○	○	○	○
Saturday	○	○	○	○	○	○	○	○	○	○	○	○	○	○	○	○	○	○	○	○	○	○	○	○
Sunday	○	○	○	○	○	○	○	○	○	○	○	○	○	○	○	○	○	○	○	○	○	○	○	○

Mood

MON
TUE
WED
THU
FRI
SAT
SUN

Daily Water Log

MON	○ ○ ○ ○ ○ ○ ○ ○
TUES	○ ○ ○ ○ ○ ○ ○ ○
WED	○ ○ ○ ○ ○ ○ ○ ○
THU	○ ○ ○ ○ ○ ○ ○ ○
FRI	○ ○ ○ ○ ○ ○ ○ ○
SAT	○ ○ ○ ○ ○ ○ ○ ○
SUN	○ ○ ○ ○ ○ ○ ○ ○

Weekly Tally & Notes

bust ------
upper arm ------
waist ------
------ **hips**
upper leg ------

Body Measurements:

BUST _____
UPPER ARM _____
WAIST _____
HIPS _____
UPPER LEG _____

Weekly Weight Tracker

CURRENT WEIGHT _____
GOAL WEIGHT _____

STRUGGLES

VICTORIES

Notes:

Decide. Commit. Succeed.

Daily Fasting Tracker

	1AM	2AM	3AM	4AM	5AM	6AM	7AM	8AM	9AM	10AM	11AM	12PM	1PM	2PM	3PM	4PM	5PM	6PM	7PM	8PM	9PM	10PM	11PM	12AM
Monday	○	○	○	○	○	○	○	○	○	○	○	○	○	○	○	○	○	○	○	○	○	○	○	○
Tuesday	○	○	○	○	○	○	○	○	○	○	○	○	○	○	○	○	○	○	○	○	○	○	○	○
Wednesday	○	○	○	○	○	○	○	○	○	○	○	○	○	○	○	○	○	○	○	○	○	○	○	○
Thursday	○	○	○	○	○	○	○	○	○	○	○	○	○	○	○	○	○	○	○	○	○	○	○	○
Friday	○	○	○	○	○	○	○	○	○	○	○	○	○	○	○	○	○	○	○	○	○	○	○	○
Saturday	○	○	○	○	○	○	○	○	○	○	○	○	○	○	○	○	○	○	○	○	○	○	○	○
Sunday	○	○	○	○	○	○	○	○	○	○	○	○	○	○	○	○	○	○	○	○	○	○	○	○

Mood

MON
TUE
WED
THU
FRI
SAT
SUN

Daily Water Log

MON	🝯 🝯 🝯 🝯 🝯 🝯 🝯 🝯
TUES	🝯 🝯 🝯 🝯 🝯 🝯 🝯 🝯
WED	🝯 🝯 🝯 🝯 🝯 🝯 🝯 🝯
THU	🝯 🝯 🝯 🝯 🝯 🝯 🝯 🝯
FRI	🝯 🝯 🝯 🝯 🝯 🝯 🝯 🝯
SAT	🝯 🝯 🝯 🝯 🝯 🝯 🝯 🝯
SUN	🝯 🝯 🝯 🝯 🝯 🝯 🝯 🝯

Weekly Tally & Notes

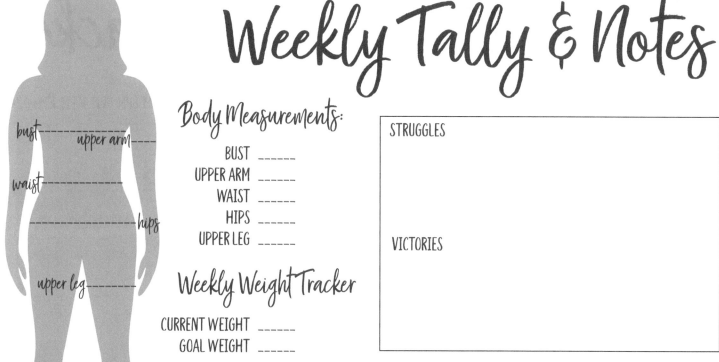

bust - - - - - - - - - -
upper arm - - - -
waist - - - - - - - - -
hips
upper leg - - - - - - -

Body Measurements:

BUST _____
UPPER ARM _____
WAIST _____
HIPS _____
UPPER LEG _____

Weekly Weight Tracker

CURRENT WEIGHT _____
GOAL WEIGHT _____

STRUGGLES

VICTORIES

Notes:

Everyday is a fresh start.

Daily Fasting Tracker

	1AM	2AM	3AM	4AM	5AM	6AM	7AM	8AM	9AM	10AM	11AM	12PM	1PM	2PM	3PM	4PM	5PM	6PM	7PM	8PM	9PM	10PM	11PM	12AM
Monday	○	○	○	○	○	○	○	○	○	○	○	○	○	○	○	○	○	○	○	○	○	○	○	○
Tuesday	○	○	○	○	○	○	○	○	○	○	○	○	○	○	○	○	○	○	○	○	○	○	○	○
Wednesday	○	○	○	○	○	○	○	○	○	○	○	○	○	○	○	○	○	○	○	○	○	○	○	○
Thursday	○	○	○	○	○	○	○	○	○	○	○	○	○	○	○	○	○	○	○	○	○	○	○	○
Friday	○	○	○	○	○	○	○	○	○	○	○	○	○	○	○	○	○	○	○	○	○	○	○	○
Saturday	○	○	○	○	○	○	○	○	○	○	○	○	○	○	○	○	○	○	○	○	○	○	○	○
Sunday	○	○	○	○	○	○	○	○	○	○	○	○	○	○	○	○	○	○	○	○	○	○	○	○

Mood

MON
TUE
WED
THU
FRI
SAT
SUN

Daily Water Log

MON	○ ○ ○ ○ ○ ○ ○ ○
TUES	○ ○ ○ ○ ○ ○ ○ ○
WED	○ ○ ○ ○ ○ ○ ○ ○
THU	○ ○ ○ ○ ○ ○ ○ ○
FRI	○ ○ ○ ○ ○ ○ ○ ○
SAT	○ ○ ○ ○ ○ ○ ○ ○
SUN	○ ○ ○ ○ ○ ○ ○ ○

Weekly Tally & Notes

bust
upper arm
waist
hips
upper leg

Body Measurements:

BUST _____
UPPER ARM _____
WAIST _____
HIPS _____
UPPER LEG _____

Weekly Weight Tracker

CURRENT WEIGHT _____
GOAL WEIGHT _____

STRUGGLES

VICTORIES

Notes:

Great things never came from comfort zones.

Daily Fasting Tracker

	1AM	2AM	3AM	4AM	5AM	6AM	7AM	8AM	9AM	10AM	11AM	12PM	1PM	2PM	3PM	4PM	5PM	6PM	7PM	8PM	9PM	10PM	11PM	12AM
Monday	○	○	○	○	○	○	○	○	○	○	○	○	○	○	○	○	○	○	○	○	○	○	○	○
Tuesday	○	○	○	○	○	○	○	○	○	○	○	○	○	○	○	○	○	○	○	○	○	○	○	○
Wednesday	○	○	○	○	○	○	○	○	○	○	○	○	○	○	○	○	○	○	○	○	○	○	○	○
Thursday	○	○	○	○	○	○	○	○	○	○	○	○	○	○	○	○	○	○	○	○	○	○	○	○
Friday	○	○	○	○	○	○	○	○	○	○	○	○	○	○	○	○	○	○	○	○	○	○	○	○
Saturday	○	○	○	○	○	○	○	○	○	○	○	○	○	○	○	○	○	○	○	○	○	○	○	○
Sunday	○	○	○	○	○	○	○	○	○	○	○	○	○	○	○	○	○	○	○	○	○	○	○	○

Mood

MON
TUE
WED
THU
FRI
SAT
SUN

Daily Water Log

MON	〇 〇 〇 〇 〇 〇 〇 〇
TUES	〇 〇 〇 〇 〇 〇 〇 〇
WED	〇 〇 〇 〇 〇 〇 〇 〇
THU	〇 〇 〇 〇 〇 〇 〇 〇
FRI	〇 〇 〇 〇 〇 〇 〇 〇
SAT	〇 〇 〇 〇 〇 〇 〇 〇
SUN	〇 〇 〇 〇 〇 〇 〇 〇

Weekly Tally & Notes

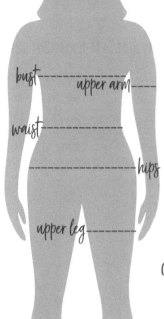

bust
upper arm
waist
hips
upper leg

Body Measurements:

BUST _____
UPPER ARM _____
WAIST _____
HIPS _____
UPPER LEG _____

Weekly Weight Tracker

CURRENT WEIGHT _____
GOAL WEIGHT _____

STRUGGLES

VICTORIES

Notes:

What you do today can improve all your tomorrows.

Daily Fasting Tracker

	1AM	2AM	3AM	4AM	5AM	6AM	7AM	8AM	9AM	10AM	11AM	12PM	1PM	2PM	3PM	4PM	5PM	6PM	7PM	8PM	9PM	10PM	11PM	12AM
Monday	○	○	○	○	○	○	○	○	○	○	○	○	○	○	○	○	○	○	○	○	○	○	○	○
Tuesday	○	○	○	○	○	○	○	○	○	○	○	○	○	○	○	○	○	○	○	○	○	○	○	○
Wednesday	○	○	○	○	○	○	○	○	○	○	○	○	○	○	○	○	○	○	○	○	○	○	○	○
Thursday	○	○	○	○	○	○	○	○	○	○	○	○	○	○	○	○	○	○	○	○	○	○	○	○
Friday	○	○	○	○	○	○	○	○	○	○	○	○	○	○	○	○	○	○	○	○	○	○	○	○
Saturday	○	○	○	○	○	○	○	○	○	○	○	○	○	○	○	○	○	○	○	○	○	○	○	○
Sunday	○	○	○	○	○	○	○	○	○	○	○	○	○	○	○	○	○	○	○	○	○	○	○	○

Mood

MON
TUE
WED
THU
FRI
SAT
SUN

Daily Water Log

MON	○ ○ ○ ○ ○ ○ ○ ○
TUES	○ ○ ○ ○ ○ ○ ○ ○
WED	○ ○ ○ ○ ○ ○ ○ ○
THU	○ ○ ○ ○ ○ ○ ○ ○
FRI	○ ○ ○ ○ ○ ○ ○ ○
SAT	○ ○ ○ ○ ○ ○ ○ ○
SUN	○ ○ ○ ○ ○ ○ ○ ○

Weekly Tally & Notes

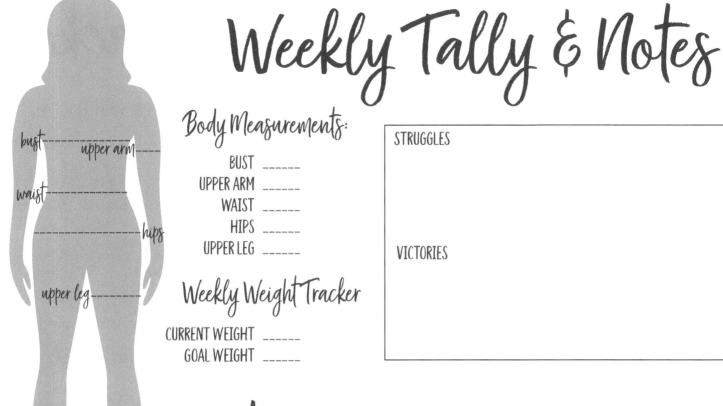

Body Measurements:

BUST _____
UPPER ARM _____
WAIST _____
HIPS _____
UPPER LEG _____

Weekly Weight Tracker

CURRENT WEIGHT _____
GOAL WEIGHT _____

STRUGGLES

VICTORIES

Notes:

Good things come to those who work for it.

Daily Fasting Tracker

	1AM	2AM	3AM	4AM	5AM	6AM	7AM	8AM	9AM	10AM	11AM	12PM	1PM	2PM	3PM	4PM	5PM	6PM	7PM	8PM	9PM	10PM	11PM	12AM
Monday	○	○	○	○	○	○	○	○	○	○	○	○	○	○	○	○	○	○	○	○	○	○	○	○
Tuesday	○	○	○	○	○	○	○	○	○	○	○	○	○	○	○	○	○	○	○	○	○	○	○	○
Wednesday	○	○	○	○	○	○	○	○	○	○	○	○	○	○	○	○	○	○	○	○	○	○	○	○
Thursday	○	○	○	○	○	○	○	○	○	○	○	○	○	○	○	○	○	○	○	○	○	○	○	○
Friday	○	○	○	○	○	○	○	○	○	○	○	○	○	○	○	○	○	○	○	○	○	○	○	○
Saturday	○	○	○	○	○	○	○	○	○	○	○	○	○	○	○	○	○	○	○	○	○	○	○	○
Sunday	○	○	○	○	○	○	○	○	○	○	○	○	○	○	○	○	○	○	○	○	○	○	○	○

Mood

MON
TUE
WED
THU
FRI
SAT
SUN

Daily Water Log

MON
TUES
WED
THU
FRI
SAT
SUN

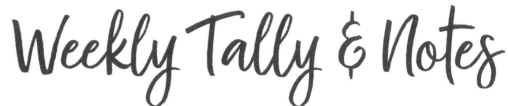

Weekly Tally & Notes

Body Measurements:

BUST	_____
UPPER ARM	_____
WAIST	_____
HIPS	_____
UPPER LEG	_____

Weekly Weight Tracker

CURRENT WEIGHT _____
GOAL WEIGHT _____

bust
upper arm
waist
hips
upper leg

STRUGGLES

VICTORIES

Notes:

You are stronger than you think.

Daily Fasting Tracker

	1AM	2AM	3AM	4AM	5AM	6AM	7AM	8AM	9AM	10AM	11AM	12PM	1PM	2PM	3PM	4PM	5PM	6PM	7PM	8PM	9PM	10PM	11PM	12AM
Monday	○	○	○	○	○	○	○	○	○	○	○	○	○	○	○	○	○	○	○	○	○	○	○	○
Tuesday	○	○	○	○	○	○	○	○	○	○	○	○	○	○	○	○	○	○	○	○	○	○	○	○
Wednesday	○	○	○	○	○	○	○	○	○	○	○	○	○	○	○	○	○	○	○	○	○	○	○	○
Thursday	○	○	○	○	○	○	○	○	○	○	○	○	○	○	○	○	○	○	○	○	○	○	○	○
Friday	○	○	○	○	○	○	○	○	○	○	○	○	○	○	○	○	○	○	○	○	○	○	○	○
Saturday	○	○	○	○	○	○	○	○	○	○	○	○	○	○	○	○	○	○	○	○	○	○	○	○
Sunday	○	○	○	○	○	○	○	○	○	○	○	○	○	○	○	○	○	○	○	○	○	○	○	○

Mood

MON
TUE
WED
THU
FRI
SAT
SUN

Daily Water Log

MON	💧 💧 💧 💧 💧 💧 💧 💧
TUES	💧 💧 💧 💧 💧 💧 💧 💧
WED	💧 💧 💧 💧 💧 💧 💧 💧
THU	💧 💧 💧 💧 💧 💧 💧 💧
FRI	💧 💧 💧 💧 💧 💧 💧 💧
SAT	💧 💧 💧 💧 💧 💧 💧 💧
SUN	💧 💧 💧 💧 💧 💧 💧 💧

Weekly Tally & Notes

Body Measurements:

BUST	_____
UPPER ARM	_____
WAIST	_____
HIPS	_____
UPPER LEG	_____

Weekly Weight Tracker

CURRENT WEIGHT	_____
GOAL WEIGHT	_____

bust _____

upper arm _____

waist _____

hips _____

upper leg _____

STRUGGLES

VICTORIES

Notes:

Your only limit is you.

Daily Fasting Tracker

	1AM	2AM	3AM	4AM	5AM	6AM	7AM	8AM	9AM	10AM	11AM	12PM	1PM	2PM	3PM	4PM	5PM	6PM	7PM	8PM	9PM	10PM	11PM	12AM
Monday	○	○	○	○	○	○	○	○	○	○	○	○	○	○	○	○	○	○	○	○	○	○	○	○
Tuesday	○	○	○	○	○	○	○	○	○	○	○	○	○	○	○	○	○	○	○	○	○	○	○	○
Wednesday	○	○	○	○	○	○	○	○	○	○	○	○	○	○	○	○	○	○	○	○	○	○	○	○
Thursday	○	○	○	○	○	○	○	○	○	○	○	○	○	○	○	○	○	○	○	○	○	○	○	○
Friday	○	○	○	○	○	○	○	○	○	○	○	○	○	○	○	○	○	○	○	○	○	○	○	○
Saturday	○	○	○	○	○	○	○	○	○	○	○	○	○	○	○	○	○	○	○	○	○	○	○	○
Sunday	○	○	○	○	○	○	○	○	○	○	○	○	○	○	○	○	○	○	○	○	○	○	○	○

Mood

MON
TUE
WED
THU
FRI
SAT
SUN

Daily Water Log

MON
TUES
WED
THU
FRI
SAT
SUN

Weekly Tally & Notes

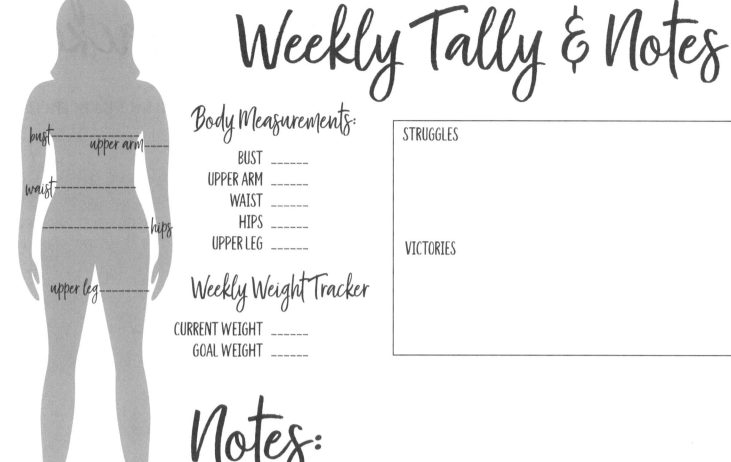

Body Measurements:

BUST _____
UPPER ARM _____
WAIST _____
HIPS _____
UPPER LEG _____

Weekly Weight Tracker

CURRENT WEIGHT _____
GOAL WEIGHT _____

STRUGGLES

VICTORIES

Notes:

Inhale the future, exhale the past.

Daily Fasting Tracker

	1AM	2AM	3AM	4AM	5AM	6AM	7AM	8AM	9AM	10AM	11AM	12PM	1PM	2PM	3PM	4PM	5PM	6PM	7PM	8PM	9PM	10PM	11PM	12AM
Monday	○	○	○	○	○	○	○	○	○	○	○	○	○	○	○	○	○	○	○	○	○	○	○	○
Tuesday	○	○	○	○	○	○	○	○	○	○	○	○	○	○	○	○	○	○	○	○	○	○	○	○
Wednesday	○	○	○	○	○	○	○	○	○	○	○	○	○	○	○	○	○	○	○	○	○	○	○	○
Thursday	○	○	○	○	○	○	○	○	○	○	○	○	○	○	○	○	○	○	○	○	○	○	○	○
Friday	○	○	○	○	○	○	○	○	○	○	○	○	○	○	○	○	○	○	○	○	○	○	○	○
Saturday	○	○	○	○	○	○	○	○	○	○	○	○	○	○	○	○	○	○	○	○	○	○	○	○
Sunday	○	○	○	○	○	○	○	○	○	○	○	○	○	○	○	○	○	○	○	○	○	○	○	○

Mood

MON
TUE
WED
THU
FRI
SAT
SUN

Daily Water Log

MON
TUES
WED
THU
FRI
SAT
SUN

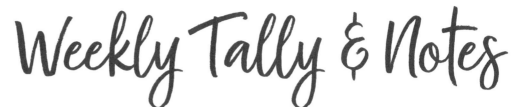

Weekly Tally & Notes

Body Measurements:

BUST _____
UPPER ARM _____
WAIST _____
HIPS _____
UPPER LEG _____

Weekly Weight Tracker

CURRENT WEIGHT _____
GOAL WEIGHT _____

STRUGGLES

VICTORIES

Notes:

bust

upper arm

waist

hips

upper leg

Strive for progress not perfection.

Daily Fasting Tracker

	1AM	2AM	3AM	4AM	5AM	6AM	7AM	8AM	9AM	10AM	11AM	12PM	1PM	2PM	3PM	4PM	5PM	6PM	7PM	8PM	9PM	10PM	11PM	12AM
Monday	○	○	○	○	○	○	○	○	○	○	○	○	○	○	○	○	○	○	○	○	○	○	○	○
Tuesday	○	○	○	○	○	○	○	○	○	○	○	○	○	○	○	○	○	○	○	○	○	○	○	○
Wednesday	○	○	○	○	○	○	○	○	○	○	○	○	○	○	○	○	○	○	○	○	○	○	○	○
Thursday	○	○	○	○	○	○	○	○	○	○	○	○	○	○	○	○	○	○	○	○	○	○	○	○
Friday	○	○	○	○	○	○	○	○	○	○	○	○	○	○	○	○	○	○	○	○	○	○	○	○
Saturday	○	○	○	○	○	○	○	○	○	○	○	○	○	○	○	○	○	○	○	○	○	○	○	○
Sunday	○	○	○	○	○	○	○	○	○	○	○	○	○	○	○	○	○	○	○	○	○	○	○	○

Mood

MON
TUE
WED
THU
FRI
SAT
SUN

Daily Water Log

MON	○ ○ ○ ○ ○ ○ ○ ○
TUES	○ ○ ○ ○ ○ ○ ○ ○
WED	○ ○ ○ ○ ○ ○ ○ ○
THU	○ ○ ○ ○ ○ ○ ○ ○
FRI	○ ○ ○ ○ ○ ○ ○ ○
SAT	○ ○ ○ ○ ○ ○ ○ ○
SUN	○ ○ ○ ○ ○ ○ ○ ○

Weekly Tally & Notes

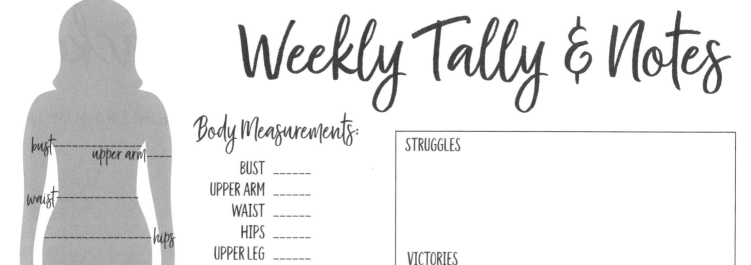

Body Measurements:

BUST _____
UPPER ARM _____
WAIST _____
HIPS _____
UPPER LEG _____

Weekly Weight Tracker

CURRENT WEIGHT _____
GOAL WEIGHT _____

STRUGGLES

VICTORIES

Notes:

You are what you do, not what you say you'll do.

WEEK FORTY EIGHT
FASTING SCHEDULE : __/__

Daily Fasting Tracker

	1AM	2AM	3AM	4AM	5AM	6AM	7AM	8AM	9AM	10AM	11AM	12PM	1PM	2PM	3PM	4PM	5PM	6PM	7PM	8PM	9PM	10PM	11PM	12AM
Monday	○	○	○	○	○	○	○	○	○	○	○	○	○	○	○	○	○	○	○	○	○	○	○	○
Tuesday	○	○	○	○	○	○	○	○	○	○	○	○	○	○	○	○	○	○	○	○	○	○	○	○
Wednesday	○	○	○	○	○	○	○	○	○	○	○	○	○	○	○	○	○	○	○	○	○	○	○	○
Thursday	○	○	○	○	○	○	○	○	○	○	○	○	○	○	○	○	○	○	○	○	○	○	○	○
Friday	○	○	○	○	○	○	○	○	○	○	○	○	○	○	○	○	○	○	○	○	○	○	○	○
Saturday	○	○	○	○	○	○	○	○	○	○	○	○	○	○	○	○	○	○	○	○	○	○	○	○
Sunday	○	○	○	○	○	○	○	○	○	○	○	○	○	○	○	○	○	○	○	○	○	○	○	○

Mood

Daily Water Log

Weekly Tally & Notes

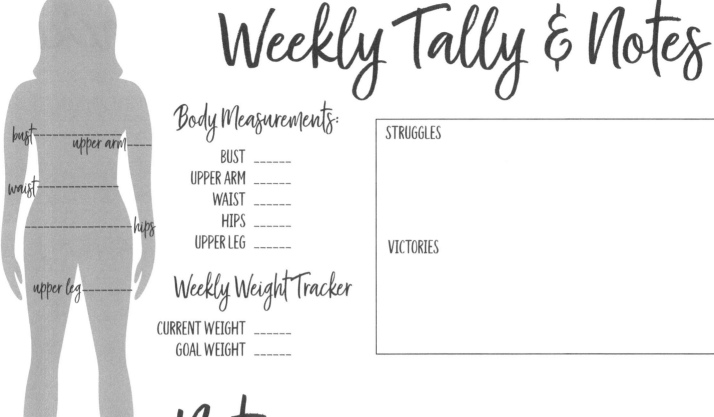

Body Measurements:

BUST _____
UPPER ARM _____
WAIST _____
HIPS _____
UPPER LEG _____

Weekly Weight Tracker

CURRENT WEIGHT _____
GOAL WEIGHT _____

STRUGGLES

VICTORIES

Notes:

You get what you work for, not what you wish for.

Daily Fasting Tracker

	1AM	2AM	3AM	4AM	5AM	6AM	7AM	8AM	9AM	10AM	11AM	12PM	1PM	2PM	3PM	4PM	5PM	6PM	7PM	8PM	9PM	10PM	11PM	12AM
Monday	○	○	○	○	○	○	○	○	○	○	○	○	○	○	○	○	○	○	○	○	○	○	○	○
Tuesday	○	○	○	○	○	○	○	○	○	○	○	○	○	○	○	○	○	○	○	○	○	○	○	○
Wednesday	○	○	○	○	○	○	○	○	○	○	○	○	○	○	○	○	○	○	○	○	○	○	○	○
Thursday	○	○	○	○	○	○	○	○	○	○	○	○	○	○	○	○	○	○	○	○	○	○	○	○
Friday	○	○	○	○	○	○	○	○	○	○	○	○	○	○	○	○	○	○	○	○	○	○	○	○
Saturday	○	○	○	○	○	○	○	○	○	○	○	○	○	○	○	○	○	○	○	○	○	○	○	○
Sunday	○	○	○	○	○	○	○	○	○	○	○	○	○	○	○	○	○	○	○	○	○	○	○	○

Mood

MON
TUE
WED
THU
FRI
SAT
SUN

Daily Water Log

MON	○ ○ ○ ○ ○ ○ ○ ○
TUES	○ ○ ○ ○ ○ ○ ○ ○
WED	○ ○ ○ ○ ○ ○ ○ ○
THU	○ ○ ○ ○ ○ ○ ○ ○
FRI	○ ○ ○ ○ ○ ○ ○ ○
SAT	○ ○ ○ ○ ○ ○ ○ ○
SUN	○ ○ ○ ○ ○ ○ ○ ○

Weekly Tally & Notes

Body Measurements:

BUST	_____
UPPER ARM	_____
WAIST	_____
HIPS	_____
UPPER LEG	_____

Weekly Weight Tracker

CURRENT WEIGHT	_____
GOAL WEIGHT	_____

STRUGGLES

VICTORIES

Notes:

It doesn't get easier. You just get stronger.

bust

upper arm

waist

hips

upper leg

Daily Fasting Tracker

	1AM	2AM	3AM	4AM	5AM	6AM	7AM	8AM	9AM	10AM	11AM	12PM	1PM	2PM	3PM	4PM	5PM	6PM	7PM	8PM	9PM	10PM	11PM	12AM
Monday	○	○	○	○	○	○	○	○	○	○	○	○	○	○	○	○	○	○	○	○	○	○	○	○
Tuesday	○	○	○	○	○	○	○	○	○	○	○	○	○	○	○	○	○	○	○	○	○	○	○	○
Wednesday	○	○	○	○	○	○	○	○	○	○	○	○	○	○	○	○	○	○	○	○	○	○	○	○
Thursday	○	○	○	○	○	○	○	○	○	○	○	○	○	○	○	○	○	○	○	○	○	○	○	○
Friday	○	○	○	○	○	○	○	○	○	○	○	○	○	○	○	○	○	○	○	○	○	○	○	○
Saturday	○	○	○	○	○	○	○	○	○	○	○	○	○	○	○	○	○	○	○	○	○	○	○	○
Sunday	○	○	○	○	○	○	○	○	○	○	○	○	○	○	○	○	○	○	○	○	○	○	○	○

Mood

MON
TUE
WED
THU
FRI
SAT
SUN

Daily Water Log

MON
TUES
WED
THU
FRI
SAT
SUN

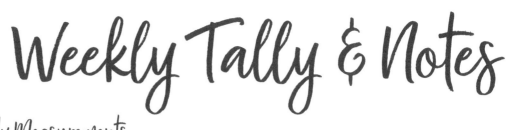

Weekly Tally & Notes

Body Measurements:

BUST _____
UPPER ARM _____
WAIST _____
HIPS _____
UPPER LEG _____

Weekly Weight Tracker

CURRENT WEIGHT _____
GOAL WEIGHT _____

STRUGGLES

VICTORIES

Notes:

Let your dreams be your wings.

Daily Fasting Tracker

	1AM	2AM	3AM	4AM	5AM	6AM	7AM	8AM	9AM	10AM	11AM	12PM	1PM	2PM	3PM	4PM	5PM	6PM	7PM	8PM	9PM	10PM	11PM	12AM
Monday	○	○	○	○	○	○	○	○	○	○	○	○	○	○	○	○	○	○	○	○	○	○	○	○
Tuesday	○	○	○	○	○	○	○	○	○	○	○	○	○	○	○	○	○	○	○	○	○	○	○	○
Wednesday	○	○	○	○	○	○	○	○	○	○	○	○	○	○	○	○	○	○	○	○	○	○	○	○
Thursday	○	○	○	○	○	○	○	○	○	○	○	○	○	○	○	○	○	○	○	○	○	○	○	○
Friday	○	○	○	○	○	○	○	○	○	○	○	○	○	○	○	○	○	○	○	○	○	○	○	○
Saturday	○	○	○	○	○	○	○	○	○	○	○	○	○	○	○	○	○	○	○	○	○	○	○	○
Sunday	○	○	○	○	○	○	○	○	○	○	○	○	○	○	○	○	○	○	○	○	○	○	○	○

Mood

MON
TUE
WED
THU
FRI
SAT
SUN

Daily Water Log

MON	◊ ◊ ◊ ◊ ◊ ◊ ◊ ◊
TUES	◊ ◊ ◊ ◊ ◊ ◊ ◊ ◊
WED	◊ ◊ ◊ ◊ ◊ ◊ ◊ ◊
THU	◊ ◊ ◊ ◊ ◊ ◊ ◊ ◊
FRI	◊ ◊ ◊ ◊ ◊ ◊ ◊ ◊
SAT	◊ ◊ ◊ ◊ ◊ ◊ ◊ ◊
SUN	◊ ◊ ◊ ◊ ◊ ◊ ◊ ◊

Weekly Tally & Notes

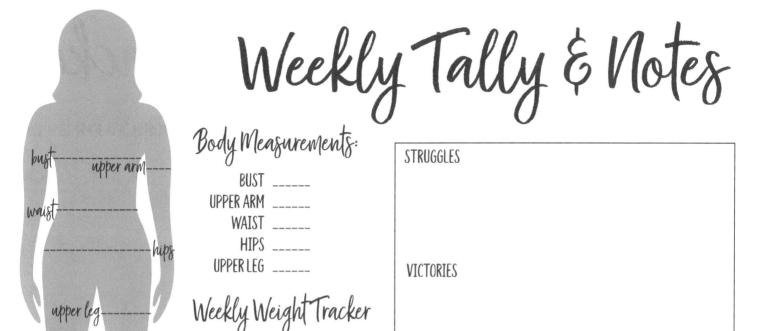

Body Measurements:

BUST _____
UPPER ARM _____
WAIST _____
HIPS _____
UPPER LEG _____

Weekly Weight Tracker

CURRENT WEIGHT _____
GOAL WEIGHT _____

STRUGGLES

VICTORIES

Notes:

Find joy in the journey.

Daily Fasting Tracker

	1AM	2AM	3AM	4AM	5AM	6AM	7AM	8AM	9AM	10AM	11AM	12PM	1PM	2PM	3PM	4PM	5PM	6PM	7PM	8PM	9PM	10PM	11PM	12AM
Monday	○	○	○	○	○	○	○	○	○	○	○	○	○	○	○	○	○	○	○	○	○	○	○	○
Tuesday	○	○	○	○	○	○	○	○	○	○	○	○	○	○	○	○	○	○	○	○	○	○	○	○
Wednesday	○	○	○	○	○	○	○	○	○	○	○	○	○	○	○	○	○	○	○	○	○	○	○	○
Thursday	○	○	○	○	○	○	○	○	○	○	○	○	○	○	○	○	○	○	○	○	○	○	○	○
Friday	○	○	○	○	○	○	○	○	○	○	○	○	○	○	○	○	○	○	○	○	○	○	○	○
Saturday	○	○	○	○	○	○	○	○	○	○	○	○	○	○	○	○	○	○	○	○	○	○	○	○
Sunday	○	○	○	○	○	○	○	○	○	○	○	○	○	○	○	○	○	○	○	○	○	○	○	○

Mood

MON

TUE

WED

THU

FRI

SAT

SUN

Daily Water Log

MON

TUES

WED

THU

FRI

SAT

SUN

Weekly Tally & Notes

> The best view comes after the hardest climb.

Notes:

STRUGGLES

VICTORIES

Body Measurements:

----- BUST
----- UPPER ARM
----- WAIST
----- HIPS
----- UPPER LEG

Weekly Weight Tracker

----- CURRENT WEIGHT
----- GOAL WEIGHT

upper leg
hips
waist
upper arm
bust

Year in Review

STARTING WEIGHT

ENDING WEIGHT

TOTAL WEIGHT LOST

TOTAL INCHES LOST

GREATEST STRUGGLE

GREATEST VICTORY

DID YOU MEET YOUR GOAL

WHAT IS YOUR NEXT GOAL

Congrats on completing an entire year of Intermittent Fasting!